Getting In

How To Stand Out From The Crowd
And Ace Your Residency Interview

Myers R. Hurt III, MD

This book is not intended to replace the services of your academic advisors or any other professionals. This book is also not a substitute for professional or legal advice. You are advised to consult with your dean's office concerning matters relating to your specific situation entering the NRMP Match.

Names of individuals and hospitals are not based on existing institutions and are provided as examples only. Any similarities to any existing institutions are purely coincidental.

Information included in this document is subject to change without notice. The author and publisher are not liable for errors or omissions appearing in this document.

ISBN: 978-0-9975955-1-2

To my former, current, and future medical students: you will all make incredible physicians.

Table of Contents

Introduction — v

PART ONE: PREPARATION — 2

Rule #1: The Program Coordinator is Your Best Friend — 2

Rule #2: Know Your Goal — 22

Rule #3: Do Your Homework — 25

Rule #4: You Are Always Being Interviewed — 30

Rule #5: Be Yourself — 32

PART TWO: INTERVIEW DAY — 35

The Day Before the Interview — 35

The Resident Dinner — 37

The Day of the Interview — 42

What are the different types of interviews? — 51

Who is interviewing you? — 54

Categories of Questions — 58

PART THREE: THE AFTERMATH — 99

Interpreting Communication Nuances — 102

Writing the Perfect Thank You Note — 104

How to Ask Follow-Up Questions — 107

Final Pearls — 111

References — 114

Introduction

Medical school is full of books by two hundred contributing authors sporting three-figure price tags. We all watch them collect dust, only to be rendered obsolete in twelve months when a new, cutting edge book is released. I wanted to buck this trend and write an accessible, no-nonsense guide to the residency interview filled with bare-bones, concise action steps students could use to better their chances in the National Residency Matching Program (NRMP) Main Residency Match (otherwise known as "the Match") now.

I successfully navigated this process myself as an applicant, matched at my number one ranked program, and then sat on the hiring side of the desk as a Chief Resident just three years later. During my tenure in academic medicine, I have personally conducted hundreds of residency interviews, read hundreds of applications, and helped applicants from both US and foreign schools successfully match into both residency and fellowship programs. The goal of this book is to give you practical interview advice that you can use today from someone who has been on both sides of the desk.

Like most aspects of medical training, the NRMP Match is an evolving process that can and will change in the future. While the data presented in this volume are properly referenced, most of the information is my opinion and reflects only my personal beliefs, not those of my former, current, or future employers. It is an opinion, however, that is firmly rooted in many years of personal experience, the experiences of my colleagues, and the experiences of my former students.

Almost all of these aforementioned students shared an annual cyclic anxiety of the interview season. Each year, each individual student would ask similar questions and I would happily give similar answers across the board. No matter the specialty, the program, or the unique circumstances you think only apply to you - common threads are shared by every successful applicant.

Balancing out those common successful traits are the common misconceptions about the matching process itself. In fact, since its introduction in 1952, the NRMP Match has been cloaked in mystery and doubt. This book is designed to help you replace speculation and rumor with facts and structure in order to tip the odds in your favor. While some of the speculation and rumors you hear are indeed true, the process itself can be straightforward, and I will help you polish the variables that you control.

The strongest variable that you control is your USMLE scores. As such, most commercially available resources involving the transition between medical school and residency placement focus solely on USMLE test preparation. Question banks, review books, flashcards, and review courses all feed multimillion dollar operations. I happily paid my fair share to these "new" pillars of medicine, and I'm sure many of you have done the same. Did you ever consider, though, why graduating physicians go through a lengthy "Match" process at all? Why is the almighty USMLE Step 1 score not a stand alone selection factor? Read on.

While no one can argue that the emphasis placed on USMLE scores is appropriate, residency program directors would maintain that the same amount of emphasis should also apply to each additional aspect of your application.

For proof, you simply need to go to the NRMP themselves.

Every two years, the NRMP sends surveys to program directors after Match Day. This data is then freely and publicly available on their website (www.NRMP.org). While USMLE Step 1 scores are consistently the number one factor in deciding which applicants to invite for interviews, those same test scores fall to number *FIVE* when deciding which of those applicants to rank and ultimately hire. Essentially, the NRMP's data tells you what to focus on to rank highly at your dream program.

The four qualities program directors value over standardized test scores across all specialties are, in order:

- Interactions with faculty during interview and visit
- Interpersonal skills
- Interactions with housestaff during interview and visit, and
- Feedback from current residents

All four of these qualities revolve around communication skills demonstrated to a handful of people in a handful of hours. This book will help you be your best self during that crucial time. The book is structured chronologically, from the interview invitations to the post-interview communication, and is peppered with quotes from former students and examples on how to specifically communicate with programs. If you are just starting the interview process, I recommend you read it through from start to finish. If you are only looking for advice about specific scenarios, however, feel free to jump to the individual topics.

After turning the last page, you will have read the only available guide that addresses the logistics, planning, psychology, and nuances specific to the residency interview. Enjoy!

PART ONE:

PREPARATION

"Proper planning and preparation prevents piss poor performance."

- *"The 7 Ps"*, United States Marine Corps

PART ONE: PREPARATION

First and foremost, there are only five simple rules to success in residency interviews:

> Rule #1: The program coordinator is your best friend
>
> Rule #2: Know your goal
>
> Rule #3: Do your homework
>
> Rule #4: You are always being interviewed
>
> Rule #5: Be yourself

Rule #1: The Program Coordinator is Your Best Friend

Only a small team of people have initial access to the flood of applications each year. At a minimum, this team consists of a Program Director (an attending physician who has clinical, research, educational, and administrative duties) and a Program Coordinator (an administrative assistant to the program director who exclusively deals with the details of the residency program. These details include recruitment, international visa issues, licensing deadlines, accreditation agreements, rotation scheduling, residency alumni, and new applicant logistics. Occasionally, a small handful of other individuals see applications at this stage. Some programs have an Assistant Program Director, a small resident recruitment committee, or perhaps one other administrative assistant to help organize data.

The importance of the program coordinators as a group is that they are in the "inner circle," even in the smallest of programs. They are THE front line in this process and your go-to contact person throughout interview season. They work closely with the program director to facilitate the recruitment process, and they look after most of the correspondence with applicants. Program coordinators communicate with applicants daily and help insulate the program director from having to answer the same questions hundreds of times.

In addition to the obviously close relationship program coordinators have with their own program directors, they are friendly with the coordinators of other residency and fellowship programs within the same hospital system, geographic region, and specialty. There are national organizations dedicated to these individuals in each specialty. One example of such an organization is the Association of Residency Coordinators in Orthopedic Surgery (ARCOS). These professional groups often meet annually, network amongst themselves and form relationships that cross state lines. Coordinators in Connecticut are on committees with those in Oregon, and coordinators in Oklahoma may have friends in Maine they can call for applicant information, both positive and negative. It behooves you a great deal to keep these people happy. Ipso facto, Rule #1 - *The program coordinator is your best friend.*

Treating these people with respect, communicating with them in a professional, polite, timely manner, and developing a positive rapport early on will help you tremendously. Conversely, any abuse of this relationship, and especially any rude behavior or offensive action directed at a program coordinator, goes straight to the program director and can affect you for years.

In short, how you interact with the program coordinator can make or break your career.

Interview Invitations:

If you have followed your medical school's advice on timelines for application submission, and assuming you have successfully navigated ERAS, FREIDA, AAMC, OASIS, ECFMG (for you International Medical Graduates (IMGs)), the NRMP, and the other swamps of medical alphabet soup, invitations to interview start rolling in soon after you submit your application.

Interview invitations will come in the form of an e-mail to the address you provided in the *Personal Information* section of MyERAS, or will be sent to the *Message Center* portal in MyERAS (not necessarily both). Programs send any rejections via the same routes. If you are not granted an interview, most programs will send you a simple message stating just that.

It goes without saying that different programs work differently, and each program will have a particular approach to the mass of electronic information that inundates them September

15th. Specific "cutoffs" and "filters" are very real, but are rarely published and not widely discussed. Furthermore, they often evolve and depend on both the preferences of each program and the personal criteria of program directors.

The data from the 2014 NRMP Match shows that when averaged across all specialties, each program gets 856 applications, interviews 96 of these applicants, and ranks 76 for 7 spots. Percentage-wise, that translates to interview invitations being sent to only 11% of initial applicants and not even 1% of that initial applicant pool (only 9% of those who are interviewed) matching with an individual program. Seem like unrealistic numbers? Remember that the applicant pool does not only consist of allopathic US seniors. The NRMP Match pool has osteopathic doctor (DO) candidates, IMGs (with graduation dates spanning at least the last five years), and allopathic graduates who either took time off for research or are currently in preliminary or transitional years. In 2014, while there were 17,374 "traditional" US allopathic seniors, a substantial 16,896 (49% of the applicant pool) came from these other sources.

But don't get discouraged! The data above needs to be taken with a grain of salt, and does not account for an individual candidate interviewing at or ranking different programs. In addition, since programs range from one to over twenty available spots, data varies highly from program to program. Furthermore, if you are an allopathic US senior, you are at a huge advantage. The 2015 data from the NRMP shows that 94% of US allopathic

5

seniors matched successfully, and 78% of those who matched did so with one of their top three choices. The low numbers above are not presented to frighten anyone, but only to reinforce what a huge field you are in. Consider yourself lucky when you receive an interview invitation - you are already in the top 10% of the applicant pool. Congratulations are in order!

How to tease out that top 10% is no easy task, either. Put yourself in the shoes of a program director who looks at potentially 1,000+ applications each year and has to slash 90% of those immediately. Hence the previously mentioned filters and cutoffs. With almost all medical schools leaning away from overall GPAs and towards the "pass", "high pass", and "honors" system, the only tangible, objective data you have on your ERAS application is your score on the USMLE. The 2015 NRMP data reflect that this score is indeed the single most important factor in getting an interview invitation. (Therefore, any reader who bought this book before First Aid for the USMLE Step 1 needs to put it down, and go study for the boards.)

Why is this important, you ask, and what does it have to do with the interview I have next week? Well, it is vital to understand that you will be competing with candidates of a similar caliber. You scored a 260 on Step 1 and a 245 on Step 2, did some research, 100+ hours of volunteer work, and have one poster that you presented at a conference? Good for you! So does everyone else dressed in a suit sitting next to you. They got the same invitation.

What makes you a better fit at this hospital? What makes you stand out that doesn't already show on paper? THESE are the reasons programs go through an interview process. This book will help you hone the necessary skills to answer these specific questions, and turn an interview invitation into a residency position.

"Make sure to check your email every day - including your Junk mailbox. I got most invitations without a problem, but did have one that was filed as 'Spam'"

- AS, Otolaryngology

When to schedule interviews:

Interview season runs from the beginning of October until the end of January each academic year. Most interview invitations will have two or three dates for you to choose from as determined by the department (i.e. they only interview on Tuesdays and Thursdays and give you a choice of two or three different dates). Reply to these as soon as you receive them, and try to maintain your selection without changing it. Consider the staggering number of applicants (of similar qualifications) the program coordinator is dealing with. Do not stand out for the wrong reasons this early in the game.

Unbeknownst to almost all medical students, yet known all too well by program coordinators, is that scheduling applicant interviews is a massive undertaking. For three months, departments juggle faculty availability, resident availability, dinner reservations, hotel reservations, hospital tours, city tours, and many other logistical concerns while answering the same questions multiple times, and, most importantly, not compromising patient care. The financial cost and time commitment of this is enormous. In a teaching hospital, time away from resident education and time away from patient care costs real money. You should act accordingly and respect the time they spend recruiting you.

One of the best ways to respect their time is to keep a calendar and stick to it. Each time you accept an invitation, write it down, and keep track of both acceptances and rejections so that you can follow up later with any programs you have not yet heard from. Use any medium that is familiar to you - hardcopy planner, Google Calendar, Outlook, Excel, or the NRMP Match Prism Scheduling app are all good options. You will need to reference this multiple times when making travel plans, scheduling interviews, and keeping up with coursework back home.

How you chronologically order your interviews is ultimately up to you, but a few patterns are often encouraged by medical school deans. The concept of a "practice interview" is often attractive. A practice interview is an interview (usually at your home institution, or one nearby) at a program you have little to no intention of matching with. These can indeed be an excellent way to help you prepare answers to any questions you did not anticipate, as well as to get an overall feel for the flow of a typical interview day. Ideally, you would then have your "dream" program interview after two or three other interview sessions.

I can't disagree with this approach, as it works extremely well and can instill a confidence in you that can absolutely land you a job. What I do disagree with is the connotation of the word "practice." By no means should you treat any of your so-called "practice" interviews as such. Not taking the day seriously, skipping out on hospital tours, and giving careless answers are not good "practice" of what you will see in the future. Imitate the real thing, and use the opportunity to try and emulate the day you will have at your dream program. Your actions and intentions are on display, and acting unprofessionally is unacceptable. Programs don't have "practice" days where they don't rank any of the applicants seen. For them, EVERY interview is a potential employee. Each interview counts just as much as any other.

At the other end of the spectrum, some applicants worry about interviewing "too late" in the season. Go ahead and erase this from your mind. As much as I would love to back up such a statement with concrete data, there are simply no data sets comparing interview date to rank list order.

Take comfort in the fact that the Match is an annual process, programs are extremely familiar with the process, and rank lists are revisited throughout the entire season. The final rank order list is never set in stone until it is submitted by the Program Director in February, so schedule your interviews when you need to schedule them. October 1st and January 31st are equally capable of producing a successful resident applicant. Now that that is settled, how many should you schedule?

"Plan ahead your 4th year and consider taking a lighter rotation or research elective during the months that are known to have the most interviews. Ask the interns at your home institution for advice."

-SG, *Plastic Surgery*

How many interviews to schedule:

Similar to the chronological order of interviews, opinions differ on how many total interviews an applicant should schedule. We all have friends who applied to 80 programs and did not get a single interview, and friends who applied to only one program and got in. I recommend you put yourself somewhere on the bell curve between those two extremes.

The 2015 NRMP Applicant survey shows that US Seniors who were successful in matching submitted a median total of 30 applications that yielded 16 interviews, and they then attended 12. IMGs are usually coached to apply to as many programs as financially possible, skewing the data to one extreme of the bell curve mentioned in the previous paragraph. In fact, when combined with IMGs and other non-US allopathic senior applicants, the successful matching candidate had a median total of 75 applications yielding 9 interviews and attended 8. Again, take these numbers with a grain of salt, as they do not account for multiple applications and multiple interview invitations. Instead, you should interpret them to mean that you need to attend as many interviews as you need to position yourself as a strong candidate in your specialty of choice. There is no definitive answer, and much of it will depend on personality and your own peace of mind.

Some advice would be: if you are trying for a competitive speciality or school, or are a mediocre candidate, shoot for above these numbers. A stellar candidate who is aiming for a less competitive school or trying to match into one of the less competitive specialties will need fewer interviews to find a good fit. The above numbers will provide a good number to shoot for (assuming time and money allow). To IMGs in particular, I'd express the following: no matter how amazing your record is, consider yourself in the first group, and attend as many interviews as you can afford.

Scheduling Pearls:

However you decide to approach the number and timing of your interviews, there is no denying that the interview trail is a marathon, not a sprint. Some additional things to bear in mind are:

Laundry and drycleaning: you'll be wearing the same clothes multiple times in a short period of time and need quick turnaround. (These same clothes need to fit after a few months of free dinners by the way.)

Health: free meals, long road trips, and sitting on planes don't burn calories, and bags under your eyes do not give good first impressions. Exercise and rest need to be priorities.

Social commitments: you may be asked to join the residents for an informal evening after your interview day, or to attend a community event that is concurrent with your stay. Plan your travel accordingly.

Travel "cushions": trains, planes, automobiles, hotel check in and check out times all need to be accounted for, as do the inevitable travel delays. Give yourself ample time on each end of an interview for travel, and plan on arriving in and departing from your interview city multiple hours away from any scheduled commitment.

School schedule: vacation time, elective blocks, research projects, USMLE Step 2 CK, CS scheduling all still need to be in the back of your mind. Don't forget you still need to graduate medical school in order to take a residency position, and you need to stay on top of your obligations back home.

"The NRMP has an official MATCH PRISM app on both iPhone and Android platforms to help track and rate programs as you see them. The University of Wisconsin has a similar app - shop around to find one you like to help stay organized."

- SA, Family Medicine

Travel Grouping:

If you have only applied to one geographic region, you are in luck - but if you have applied to a wide variety of programs, you need to take travel time and cost into consideration. For example, an applicant based in California should strive to schedule all New England interviews together (a Boston interview on Tuesday and Vermont on Thursday for example). Give yourself 2-3 days for each program at a bare minimum, be careful not to overload, and consider the weather in the region. Winter flight delays in New England are inevitable - #Jonasblizzard.

With the right timing, you can fly into one region, and use a rental car to commute between multiple interviews in one or more cities. Scheduling locations that are a good distance from your home institution multiple weeks apart will add up quickly.

Applicants who are doing extensive traveling (i.e. IMGs or top-tier applicants applying to high caliber programs coast to coast) may want to look into credit card travel miles and travel loyalty programs. Frequent flier miles and free hotel nights can add up to a fantastic vacation after graduation. The Capital One Venture card and Chase Sapphire Preferred both have good programs at the time of this publication. More importantly, they are most valuable when a good chunk of change is spent in the first month, easily doable on the interview trail. Shop around to find the best deal based on your geographic region and airline of choice.

Getting In

"I used the travel app TripIt Pro to pull confirmation numbers and flight times straight from my email to help keep flight reservations, hotel reservations, and rental car details organized for quick access when visiting multiple programs."

- KM, General Surgery

A common "travel grouping" case involves those of you entering the match as a couple. It is completely acceptable to reach out to corresponding programs if your partner was granted an interview. Program coordinators are more than accommodating when applicants reach out to them to help coordinate these things. A potential way to approach this topic in a professional fashion is shown below:

Dear Mr. Smith,

I wanted to reach out to you and let the department know that my wife was offered a residency interview with the Radiology department on December 9th.

I have not yet heard back from your program regarding my application to your Pediatrics program, but we are entering the Couples Match, and if you were considering me for an interview, we would like to possibly coordinate interview dates.

We are both extremely interested in Denver, and would make an interview with your program a top priority.

Sincerely,

Myers Hurt

Changing Dates and Canceling Interviews:

Timing is indeed everything when changing dates or canceling interviews, and decisions need to be made as early as possible. A few schedule changes weeks in advance is appropriate, especially for travel grouping as explained above, but as the interview date approaches, consider it set in stone. These programs are recruiting you, and you should show them your appreciation by respecting their time.

If you find yourself needing to change an interview date, email is an appropriate mode of communication. You will not be the first person to reschedule an interview, nor will you be the last. Take comfort in the fact that program coordinators deal with rescheduling all the time. Every single one of them knows you are interviewing with a number of other programs, and it does not look like you are giving one program priority over another by requesting a reschedule. This will not affect your rank order in any way. Address your request to the program coordinator, and keep it concise. Example:

Mr. Smith,

I have been granted two additional interviews in Massachusetts and would like to try and keep travel costs at a minimum (I will be flying in from Nebraska). Do you have any additional available interview dates the second week of December I could reschedule into?

I understand the schedule is tight, and appreciate the effort. Looking forward to meeting you in person!

Myers Hurt

ERAS #12345

"Pro Tip: include your ERAS number in all correspondence with the department - this makes it easier for them to locate your record and identify you."

- MK, Emergency Medicine

The above rules apply to canceling interviews. Give programs ample time to fill your canceled spot with an applicant on the waiting list. Canceling is somewhat expected late in the season, as applicants either interview with enough programs to feel confident about their chances of matching, or they simply run out of allocated funds and energy. Unlike rescheduling, canceling an interview definitively shows that you are not interested. Do not expect to get a second opportunity at or to be ranked by a program you have canceled. A concise email to the program coordinator is again appropriate. Example:

Mr. Smith,

Thank you again for the opportunity to interview at XXX. Unfortunately, due to time constraints I need to cancel our scheduled interview on December 8th.

I hope it is not too much of an inconvenience, and appreciate your time.

> *Sincerely,*
> *Myers Hurt*
> *ERAS #12345*

Be sure to cancel interviews that you have no intention of attending. Neglecting to do so is unprofessional, and the knowledge of this behavior will spread from program to program. This endangers your ability to be considered elsewhere.

A former program coordinator told me of one infamous applicant who accepted interview invitations to four programs in a major city, checked into all hotels the programs paid for, and did not attend a single resident event at any of the hosting departments. That "joyride" weekend not only cost him a job through the Match, he got to spend his free time during unemployment to deal with lawsuits.

Canceling or rescheduling at the last minute for an emergency is not the end of the world. Don't miss the birth of your child for a residency interview. However, be mature and responsible about the process. Call the program coordinator to apologize and explain the situation. Do not email a last-minute cancellation; this is on par with breaking up via text message. Be an adult and talk to the coordinator.

It is also appropriate to request a reschedule if this is a "dream program," but understand this may not be a possibility.

"Don't be afraid to ask Program Coordinators advice on where to stay - I had many friends get free accommodation with a resident or medical student living close to the hospital."

- TB, Internal Medicine

There's an App for That:

Recently, new services have emerged that will soon replace the archaic system of interview scheduling. Thalamus and Interview Broker are two examples of software platforms you may encounter this interview season. They remove the burden of scheduling hundreds of interviews from program coordinators and let them focus on more human recruitment tasks. Similarly, by mirroring the hospitality models of AirBnb and Couchsurfing, a medical-student specific service known as Swap and Snooze connects fourth year students looking for a place to stay on the interview trail.

"I used Swap and Snooze to find housing at a few of my interviews. Spending time with students at those programs gave me a deeper understanding of what life would be like there."

- MG, Internal Medicine

Radio Silence:

What if I don't hear anything? Will I seem obnoxious if I email today? How many calls are too many? I applied two weeks ago and haven't heard back.

Don't panic.

Most programs are upfront about waiting until October 1st *at the earliest* so that they can include the Medical Student Performance Evaluation (MSPE) or "Dean's letter" with applications. Some programs download ERAS applications in "chunks" and simply may have not processed your application yet. Furthermore, it takes time to thoughtfully review even a "filtered" applicant pool.

Akin to the timing subtleties involved with interview scheduling, a certain etiquette applies to reaching out to a program. If you have not heard anything from a program to which you have applied, it is perfectly fine to reach out to them with an e-mail or phone call. Again, be conscious of not standing for the wrong reasons. No program coordinator likes fielding thirty-seven frantic calls from an overzealous applicant, but if you are concerned, saying something is appropriate.

For an application submitted immediately on September 15th, four to six weeks is a reasonable amount of time to wait before contacting departments. If you applied later in the season, however (say late November,) a follow up call or e-mail in just two weeks is fine.

Communicate only with the program coordinator. Emailing the program director directly or even cc'ing them on your correspondence is not the best idea unless you know them personally (i.e. you rotated with them and made a strong, positive impression). Another good option for a direct line to a program director is for one of your faculty advisors or mentors to call and put in the proverbial "good word" for you.

Example:

Dear Mr. Smith,

I have not yet heard from your program regarding my application to your residency program. I am extremely interested in XXX and if invited would make an interview with your program my top priority. Please let me know if there are any discrepancies in my application I can help clear up.

Sincerely,

Myers Hurt

ERAS #12345

IMG Pearl - On average, you will be applying to a much larger number of programs over multiple time zones. It will be beneficial to make a spreadsheet of the programs you have and haven't heard back from, as well as contact numbers. Skype and MagicJack (with a US number) are the best options for making international calls to the US to correspond with program coordinators. For you, Rule #1 applies tenfold.

Social Media Considerations:

Generation Y, millennials, echo boomers...whatever name sticks, you are part of a generation that has never known life without the Internet. Your generation grew up with social media. Playground fights previously witnessed by only a few now end up on Worldstar; encyclopedias that previously filled libraries are now at our fingertips. And we all know what Kim Kardashian looks like naked. Great.

As a future physician, what you need to know about social media is this: don't post anything on any platform that is of questionable content. If you are a decent human being with little to no formal criminal record, this is probably already the case - but it goes a bit deeper than that.

I highly doubt any program director or program coordinator will personally search for an applicant's name "just to see what pops up". In addition, I highly doubt ERAS will be adding a link to your Instagram account anytime soon. (That is, unless they can find a way to charge us yet another fee for it)

What *is* a possibility, however, and a much more likely scenario, is a resident Googling an applicant name. Residents are exposed to only a fraction of the applicant pool at social events, dinners, and the occasional interview, and may be curious to look up what is publically available. In addition, they are more familiar with social media platforms than the *ahem*..."more distinguished" attendings, and would probably be more inclined to type in an applicant name. If you are attractive, they absolutely will.

The short-term solution to the "social media problem" is to change your real name during the interview season on sites like Facebook, Instagram and Twitter during the interview season. Make sure your privacy settings are where you want them. There is no need to disable your account completely. Long-term, it's of course always a good idea to refrain from posting keg-stand pics in a thong. After all, you have another round of interviews for fellowships or "real" jobs after residency.

"You hold an NCAA record for Jager bombs and streaked homecoming three years in a row? Awesome - they will be great pics for your residency graduation roast - but they won't help get you there."

- OB, *General Surgery*

Rule #2: Know Your Goal

Your goal is to get a job, period. It is important to remember this, as a job interview is very different from the academic interviews you have had in the past. Form the proper mindset when embarking on the interview trail, and develop a game plan.

In the "real world" (read: nonmedical), a poor hire costs a company money. A poor hire may be slow to train, abuse company resources, or unable to effectively close deals. In medicine, and more specifically, at the exact transition from med school to residency, the stakes are much higher. A poor hire can potentially cost patient lives. Residency programs are aware of this, and interview accordingly.

To meet the unique needs of hiring residents, the interview has been constructed accordingly. This process is one part academic interview, one part job interview, and one part first date all rolled into one. Programs have four to six hours to glean information about you that can not be objectively quantified, or written on paper. Essentially, they have only a handful of hours to get a "gut feel" for an applicant.

Psychologically, you need to prepare yourself to deliver a crisp, clear message that you are the right applicant for the job. And remember: it is just that, a job.

First and foremost, it is imperative that you realize that you are qualified for the job. As mentioned before, you will be going up against applicants of a similar caliber (at least objectively). You have worked hard, cleared hurdles, made the cutoffs and filters, and impressed people enough to be sitting in the interview chair. Be proud of yourself! As much as you want to impress the department in order to get a residency position, they want to impress applicants in order to attract top talent. In fact, interviewers are trained to serve as ambassadors to their respective programs.

We can see this relationship by again turning to the NRMP data, and looking this time at the *Applicant Survey* instead of the *Program Director's Survey*. The 2015 NRMP *Applicant Survey* shows that the most important factors applicants considered when *applying* to programs were "geographic location" and "reputation of program." When asked why those chose to *rank* a program, however, the top factors were "overall goodness of fit" and "interview day experience" across all specialties. See how residency interviews are clearly a two way street? Part of your goal in framing your mindset is to realize that you are also interviewing them. You need to see if this program is up to the high standards you hold yourself to. Outstanding applicants have outstanding options, and hospitals will be working hard to recruit the best and the brightest; knowing this should give you some degree of comfort.

In fact, hospitals have great incentive to fill all of their available spots in the Match. Hard to believe, perhaps, but programs who do not impress enough candidates or make poor ranking decisions run the risk of exhausting their rank order list without filling all of their open residency spots. Not only does this reflect poorly on the the program and staff, the program can actually lose money, as a majority of resident salary is funded by Medicare expecting patient care in return. Not filling all available spots can result in a mandated smaller program the following year. Hence the quagmire that is the Post-Match Supplemental Offer and Acceptance Program (SOAP), previously known as the "Scramble" (a much better term for it). That is a topic for another day, but rest assured, they are wooing you.

Putting yourself in the position of "interviewer" as opposed to "interviewee" is a powerful psychological tool that can make you come across as confident, informed, and motivated. You can align your questions and answers to the goals of the program and to the individual asking them. Address their needs and desires instead of your own. How, you ask? Rule #3: Do your Homework.

Rule #3: Do Your Homework

Prior to your interview, you will be given a detailed itinerary of the interview day. I recommend listing any faculty or resident names you find on a given itinerary, and then focusing your energy on the departmental website. (We will elaborate on the interview day schedule in Rule #4.)

By gathering as much information as you can from a department website, not only will you be in a better position to discuss information during your interview, you will also reduce the amount of stress the day brings. As you may already know, being well prepared can reduce anxiety levels to the point of physically slowing your heart rate, and make you not just feel but also *look* more in control.

You can get an overall feel for the program you are interested in, and get a starting place for your questions, by visiting program web sites. All of these sites generally have department news, faculty profiles, photos of recent resident events, faculty awards, and publications. Write down questions you have, and write down specific reasons you are the best fit in each program you look into. You can come back to these notes frequently, and review them right before heading into each interview. What should you look at specifically?

Read information specific to the program: Read the program goals and vision or mission statement. If you know the specific goals of a program (a certain type of accreditation they are pursuing or a special missionary vision) you can apply it to an answer of what makes this program stand apart, and why you will be a good fit. When the program director asks "What questions do you have for me?" you can ask a well-informed question around a clarification or extrapolation of something you read. Example:

"I read that Dr. Hurt presented at the national conference last year - is there support and funding built into the department to encourage all residents to do the same?"

Or:

"The program at my home institution recently became a Patient Centered Medical Home so I am familiar with the amount of effort that takes- congrats on the recent accreditation!"

These types of questions or statements will show that you did your research, and that you are not only interested in the program now but are also thinking about the future.

Read information specific to each interviewer: Take the list you created from your itinerary and spend time gathering insight into your interviewers themselves. Ask them questions about their individual areas of interest, and use what you find online to facilitate conversation. During your time together they will be much more inclined to discuss their professional research and personal hobbies when prompted. It is perfectly acceptable to lead into a conversation with:

"Congratulations on your recent award from the ACOG! I went to the spring conference last year and would be interested in any ongoing projects."

Or even:

"I read on the department website that you enjoy fly fishing - any spots around town you recommend?"

Read information specific to the specialty: Look at the "American Academy of *(insert specialty here)*" websites. All specialties will have state and national associations with robust websites and print journals. If you weren't already reading them as part of a student interest group, skim these now for up to date issues in the field and be ready to talk about them. If you come across as knowledgeable on pertinent, current issues in the interviewer's field, you will demonstrate your value right off the bat. One well-crafted and well-placed statement will send a message that you spend time reading relevant material, are forward thinking, and can contribute to your group of peers.

Read information specific to medicine in general: I often recommend applicants take time to review current United States health policy as well as specific policy issues that would affect the department and the specialty. Possible topics include managed health care or the Affordable Care Act. Specialty-specific issues could be the legal issues surrounding the role of midlevel providers in rural areas (very important in Family Medicine and primary care career planning), CNAs practicing alongside or replacing anesthesiologists (obviously concerning for budding anesthesiologists), or employers preferring hand surgeons trained in orthopedic surgery programs instead of plastic surgery programs...you get the idea. Having an opinion on these and other issues that impact many (or all) medical groups and hospitals is vital for the future of your speciality of interest, and for your future personally in the case of being knowledgeable during the interview.

"When looking into general medical topics outside of textbooks, I found that the New York Times, Google Health, and KevinMD are reliable sources of information."

- RA, Internal Medicine

Read information specific to residency training: It will be very worth your time to read about the ACGME (Accreditation Council of Graduate Medical Education), and their RRCs (Residency Review Committees). The ACGME is the organization that all residency programs in every specialty are beholden to, and using jargon you pick up on their websites shows you are familiar with their policies.

For example, the "Six Core Competencies" of the ACGME are: professionalism, patient care, medical knowledge, practice-based learning, systems-based practice, and interpersonal skills. You will be evaluated in these areas over the next few years, so familiarize yourself with them and you will be ahead of the game. In addition, if a program has had any legal action taken against them, or has been on probation, the ACGME website will have this information.

You should also browse the expectations and official rules of the NRMP on their official site, along with the Main Residency Match timeline, calendar, and deadlines. Knowledge is power, and it behoves you to read and reread information straight from the proverbial horse's mouth.

Preparing with Mock Interviews:

Most US medical schools offer some type of mock interview preparation. I highly recommend utilizing these resources. Getting into the program of your dreams is the same way you get to Carnegie Hall: practice, practice, practice.

If your school does not offer these resources, it is imperative that you find someone to practice with. Ideally, anyone who has recently gone through the process would be best. Any friends you have that are now in their intern year would be the most helpful. Friends or family members are a decent backup choice. Practice answering questions confidently, and learn how to integrate details you want to include even when not directly asked.

Recording yourself - using both audio and video - can be an eye opening experience, and will show your posture, eye contact, and body language as seen from the perspective of an interviewer. Seeing yourself in action can help you identify and eliminate fidgeting, multiple "ummmmm"s, or "like"'s, and will help your words flow a bit more smoothly.

"After recording myself I saw how ridiculous I look chewing gum and bouncing my left leg up and down constantly. Small nervous ticks looked huge on film."
- SP, Internal Medicine

If you are taking anything away from this book at all, I hope that one point is becoming increasingly clear: Just because you speak English, own a nice suit, and destroyed the USMLE Step 1, you are not guaranteed anything. Don't jeopardize years of sacrifice and hard work by not preparing well. Unlike your previous interviews that granted you the opportunity to pay more money to a school for a fancy piece of paper, this is for your first REAL job in the career you have been working so hard for. Practice, practice, practice.

Rule #4: You Are Always Being Interviewed

As mentioned in the previous section, you should expect an itinerary for your interview day at least one week prior to your interview. Usually, the schedule consists of dinner the night prior to interview day, followed by interview day itself. Interview day has a traditional pattern of a light breakfast followed by a facility tour, some educational presentations about the hospital and the residency program, a handful of interviews, and a light lunch. These often conclude around 3:00 PM. The names of the faculty and residents you will be interviewing with are also included.

Do not let this beautiful outline fool you. No matter what your schedule says, and no matter who you are conversing with, you are constantly on display. This observation yields Rule #4: You are always being interviewed.

Whether you're interviewing in Buford, Wyoming or downtown Manhattan, you are equally on display for your potential new town. Not to be paranoid, but you don't know who's who in the new town. Even at your home institution, you don't know everyone. The lady in the elevator? Chair of Hematology. The guy at the hotel bar last night? Burnt-out cardiologist meeting his mistress. The guy you cut off on the way to the interview? The Chief Resident you'll meet in an hour. So, best behavior at all times...even if you think no one is paying attention. *Anyone you meet can and will have a say over your future employment.*

(FYI - the above three scenarios are taken verbatim from real life examples.)

Please don't misinterpret this advice. There is no need to go out of your way to be something you are not. There is, however no reason to act selfishly, drive erratically, or block elevator doors because this is "your" important day. The hospital will keep running with or without you.

Going out into the late hours the night before or night after your interview day is risky as well. You very well may run into people you will see the next day. Unless, of course, you look like James Bond when you sip martinis; go for it by all means in that case. I would just recommend against getting hammered with an old college friend you haven't seen in years at some trendy nightclub and making a complete ass of yourself. Be responsible.

"All of the applicants went to morning report on my interview day. I thought it was just to kill time, but two different faculty asked me about the presented case report later that day. I wish I would have paid just a little more attention!"

- SW, OB/Gyn

Rule #5: Be Yourself

FInally, after all the advice and prep work and stress, there is little you can do to change your personality. As cliched as it sounds, just be yourself. Honestly representing yourself on interview day will help you know if these are a group of people you will get along with for the next few years of your life, and it will let them know if you are a good fit with their team. No fluff or additional explanation needed here. Just be yourself.

PART TWO:

INTERVIEW DAY

"Being late is not being fifteen minutes early."
-Tom Coughlin, Head Coach, New York Giants

PART TWO: INTERVIEW DAY

The Day Before the Interview

So your type A gunner self has created the optimal interview trail, and you have perfectly timed your journey with weather patterns to ski Colorado while interviewing in Denver, hit the wine country when between interviews in San Francisco and Fresno, then finish up with foliage, apple picking, and a maple syrup farm in Vermont. Well done.

If you were paying attention to anything earlier, you made travel arrangements putting you in your interview town about 3 to 4 hours before the resident dinner. Assuming no travel delays or other hiccups, this gives you plenty of time to explore and prepare.

I am a huge fan of a "dry run." This means you should know exactly how you are going to get to the hospital the next day, and have a backup plan. If you will be driving, I recommend you drive to the interview location in daylight so you can recognize landmarks and anticipate any potential obstacle the following day. (i.e. parade signs, ongoing construction, etc.)

"Maybe a bit neurotic, but I had multiple backup plans for transportation - I knew how long it would take me to get to the interview via taxi, Uber, and public transportation."

- GM, Neurology

As you know, hospitals are huge and often consist of dozens of buildings. Residency interviews are held in academic office settings that can be located far from clinical sites, so give yourself plenty of time to find the *exact* building you will need to be at in the morning.

Feel free to clarify directions, parking information, and exact location specifics with the residents at the dinner later in the evening.

Some of the specific small but important steps to ensuring that everything goes off without a hitch include the following:

- *Have a plan.* Good stress management can involve many things. Handle this how you would a USMLE. Get good quality rest the night before, avoid alcohol and caffeine, meditate, get a massage, exercise - anything that will help you relax.

- *Lay out your outfit.* Even the best suits look foolish with no belt or mismatched socks, and you need to make sure you have everything you need. Your outfit includes two pens and folio with paper for your notes, as well as any medications or snacks you may need (think food allergy or dietary restrictions; come prepared.)

- *Set multiple alarms.* This is not the time to oversleep. Your usual cell phone alarm is best augmented by the wake-up call that is available at all hotels.

- *Personal hygiene.* Make it happen. Cut your fingernails, bathe, and make sure you have toothpaste, as tomorrow you are sitting face-to-face with your future boss.

- *Review your prep work.* Double check your interview schedule so you are prepared for the flow of the upcoming day. Review your responses to the questions you know you will be asked, and review the questions you know you want to ask (we'll cover good examples of both in the next section). Your goal is to leave the program with a taste of "who you are" with a desire to know more about you. In addition, you want to leave with the answers you need to help you choose whether or not the program is a good fit with you.

The Resident Dinner

What to expect:

Normally, the night before the interview day, a small handful of current residents will host a dinner. Usually this is at a local restaurant, and on rare occasions it can be a faculty member's home. In most programs, it is common that junior-level residents attend the dinners while senior levels conduct interviews the following day.

On average one to three junior residents attend dinners with one to five applicants. Spouses are generally allowed, but confirm with the program coordinator well in advance to make sure. Children are never allowed, and even if the program coordinator goes out of their way to tell you otherwise, leave them at home.

Early in the interview season, you will meet bright eyed and bushy tailed interns happy to be out of the hospital, and equally happy to get a free meal. As such, the dynamics of these dinners essentially put you in a room with people who were exactly where you are now (fourth-year medical student) just three short months ago.

Towards the end of the season, however, both applicants and residents usually lose their steam. Asking and answering the same question dozens of times takes its toll. I have been to plenty of interviews with the obligatory chief resident, "forced" to sit through another interview with glazed over eyes, dumping logo-emblazoned swag into the laps of applicants and grunting through rehearsed answers that are no longer unique to the situation or well thought out.

In either scenario, the residents will be very easy to approach at the dinner, and are happy to give details not necessarily divulged in a formal interview setting. There is no set "question time" or "eating time," and you should ask questions throughout the meal as you would in any other situation where you are meeting new people. It is important that you maintain enough enthusiasm to leave a good impression, and to get enough information to help you make a rank-order list decision.

What to wear:

Attire for this event needs to be professional, but does not need to be formal, and you should leave the suit for tomorrow. Think "business casual." Males should wear jeans or slacks with a collared shirt (tucked in) and leather shoes, with or without blazer for cooler weather. No sandals, no matter how "laid back" the program insists the dinner is. It is always better to dress down once you arrive instead of being unable to dress up. Females should also think "business casual" and consider jeans or khakis, nice shoes, plain blouse or cotton shirt (avoid low-cut), wear modest jewelry, and apply a modest amount of makeup. Jackets or sweaters are appropriate for cooler weather. No visible tattoos for either sex if possible. Medicine remains a "conservative" profession, even if medical school seems filled with young progressive liberals.

"Dark colors work best for jackets, pants, and skirts, as you can then accessorize shoes, scarves, belts and jewelry to add color and patterns."
- GB, Psychiatry

Even with "business casual" attire, the environment will be much more relaxed than you will experience the following day. Capitalize on this opportunity to speak more informally and more candidly with the residents (not crudely or unprofessionally, mind you). Now is the time to ask the questions that are a bit more personal, and questions that involve life outside of the hospital, as well as social dynamics inside the program. Usually answers to these types of questions are not on the website, and are not appropriate for department faculty. They are important, however, and can influence your decision to spend multiple years of your life with these people, so ask them.

What to Order:

If you are like most, you might be thinking: enough with the residents and the outfits! Tell me more about this free food situation! So much delicious food. And all free! What should I order?

To remove the stigma surrounding the cost of most dishes, some programs have a set menu with multiple options devoid of price information from which you can make a selection. If not, common sense applies. Don't order three lobster tails with endangered baby white seal steak, but at the same time, don't feel obligated to order a side salad and water. Order what you would normally order at a similar function at a modest price point.

I would recommend you keep your meal somewhat light, and free from rich, stain-potential sauces. Think of taking a first date to suck crawfish heads or tear through an all-you-can-eat BBQ buffet - not the most flattering conversation dishes. You want a dinner that is hassle free and allows you to chat while not having to tie a bib on and go for the house speed record. There is no need to be the butt of any jokes the next day (or next few years).

I would also recommend avoiding the unknown. Eat something you are familiar with. You do not want to be up all night sweating with stomach cramps, and you certainly don't want to be fidgeting and running to the bathroom every hour tomorrow. The interview trail is also not the time to find out that you are allergic to "foraged Panamanian cashew skin" or "essence of escargot", even if someone else is footing the bill.

Food allergies, vegetarianism, and food preferences are vast in the world of US medicine, and menus will be considered accordingly. Furthermore, religions abound, and programs have a mix of Christian, Hindu, Muslim, Jewish, atheist, and a host of other denominations in their resident population. The dietary restrictions enforced by all of these (halal, kosher, etc.) are widely accepted, and you should not hesitate to communicate your food preferences for fear of being judged. Restaurants know this, and more importantly program coordinators know this, and they plan accordingly.

To drink, water, juices, soft drinks, coffee and tea are all acceptable. I recommend abstaining from all alcohol while on the residency trail, however. Remember Rule #4: You are always being interviewed. No matter how much you think you know your limits, alcohol can find a way to rear its ugly head. Too many negative possibilities abound. You could say something stupid, engage in lewd behavior, or reveal too much. Even if your hosts are having wine or beer with their meals, politely declining is appropriate, and will not cost you a job.

Basic manners 101 applies to this dinner as well. No chewing with your mouth open, don't eat like you are starving, and no elbows on the table. Don't order some ridiculously rare off-menu item to sound sophisticated, and don't send any dishes back because you found a hair or it wasn't cooked perfectly. Treat the waitstaff with the utmost respect, and be polite to everyone for the entire evening. Show that you can function in a civilized environment, and be a flexible, accommodating adult.

Finally, remember the names of the residents from this meal, as well as a few key items you discussed. Tomorrow multiple people will ask you who you went to dinner with, and what you talked about. Coming across as disinterested is not a good thing, and simply remembering the names of your hosts will show programs you are serious about working with them in the future.

"Two things I never used before but used daily on the interview trail - a lint roller and a Tide stick - both come through in the clutch."

- JC, Emergency Medicine

The Day of the Interview

Be early. If by some act of God or Nature you are running late, call the program coordinator. Have their contact number on hand. Arriving to the interview late is not the end of the world, as long as you call (not email), and explain the situation in a timely manner.

It is embarrassing that it even has to be said, but come to the interview alone. Do not bring a friend, spouse, child, or your mother to the interview. The department will not be able to accommodate them, and you will look extremely unprofessional.

What to wear:

As mentioned previously, at its core medicine is still a conservative discipline. Most of the people interviewing you, with rare exception, will value a conservative appearance, even subconsciously.

I personally find it interesting that we need to look our best for the opportunity to look our worst. You'll look in the mirror halfway through your intern year and find a tired, disheveled shell of your old self in mismatched, oversized scrubs and a yellowed "white" coat with ripped pockets. Every inch of you will have stains of unknown origins that could only obtained at some sort of medical Burning Man: blood, urine, feces, Betadine, hand sanitizer, and coffee. I digress.

Applicants of all genders should be well groomed with clean haircuts, well-kept nails, and fresh breath. Wear little to no perfume or cologne, minimal jewelry, and attempt to cover all tattoos. Do not smell like cigarettes. Do not show up hungover.

The ideal outfit for males is a well-fitting two piece suit (no vest - this is not your cousin's wedding). Solid, dark colors are preferred, and navy or dark grey is best. Also appropriate are a crisp white or light blue shirt free from wrinkles or stains, and either a solid or striped tie with minimal (or no) designs. There is no need for pocket squares, tie clips, cuff links, or any other formal wear. The only acceptable jewelry for males is a watch and wedding ring. Footwear should be leather lace-up or slip-on shoes with appropriate dress socks. Hospitals want to hire *doctors*, not 1998 Dennis Rodman.

"Carry your suit with you or wear it when travelling. Every round of interviews I've seen bags lost leaving guys suitless."

-BT, *Plastic Surgery*

The ideal outfit for females is also a well-fitting two piece suit. Pant suits and skirt suits are equally appropriate. Ideal color schemes are dark grey, navy, or black with a light-colored blouse or cotton shirt. Wear minimal jewelry. A simple necklace and earrings are appropriate. Wear neutral nail polish. For shoes, a mid-heel closed toe pump is generally a safe choice. No short skirts, loud jewelry, or huge amounts of makeup.

"Be sure to wear comfortable shoes - you will be walking ALL DAY LONG and will need to keep up with tour groups."

- RJ, *Internal Medicine*

I know I told you to "be yourself" in Rule #5, and I am not trying to neutralize your colorful personality with drab attire. I would just suggest that you follow Rule #5 while wearing the above outfit. This clean, crisp, and otherwise plain look may not be in your everyday comfort zone, but it serves one purpose - to keep the focus on you. Just as food is best presented on a white plate, your words will stand out while wearing a simple and classic outfit. Allow your personality to shine through your diction and interactions, not your attire.

I'll also stress that you should wear attire along these lines even if interviewing with "quirky" or "granola" programs who tell you to dress casually or where faculty interview you in jeans and sneakers. The interviewers will appreciate your effort to look professional; it signifies that you are taking your future seriously. You can always let your "crazy flag" fly occasionally in terms of dress once you get the job. Just not today.

What to bring:

More important is what not to bring. Do not bring any backpacks, briefcases, or suitcases. All hotels will let you store bags with a concierge while you interview. Keep it simple.

You should bring only a thin leather folio. In said folio should be a pad of paper for notes, along with extra copies of your CV, personal statement, and reprints of any publications you would want your future employer to see. Having three to five copies of each should be sufficient. Yes, your interviewers already have access to most of these documents, but it does not hurt to have a copy on hand if they have a desk buried in paperwork or a computer with a slow internet connection.

Bring two good pens. The second pen serves as a backup for you, as well as a potential offering to another applicant. Simply offering a pen to someone in need can be a not-so-subtle demonstration of preparedness, teamwork, and kindness to your future employers.

Bring small, light snacks. The program will likely provide a light breakfast and lunch, but not snacks between sessions. As mentioned previously, vegetarian, kosher, and other dietary or religious restrictions are all taken into account for most meals, but those of you with food allergies or who are picky eaters may be out of luck when it comes to smaller snacks. Acting "hangry" in front of your future employers will not let them see the best side of you. Have a granola bar or other quick snack available for long tours or long periods of time between food options.

Bring medications. It is perfectly acceptable to bring any necessary medications you take to the interview day, including any scheduled pills or inhalers.

(An additional note for females, while the above items will likely fit in a jacket or pant pocket, if you must carry a purse, similar rules apply. Small, simple, solid color leather is best. No chains, giant logos, or other bells and whistles.)

"Bring Kleenex in case you sneeze...or cry - it has happened."

46

-CT, Family Medicine

How to behave:

Recall Rule #4: You are always being interviewed. Do not adopt the mindset that you are only "switched on" while interviewing with the program director, and then let your guard down for residents or between sessions. Be on your best behavior at all times.

Your behavior and interaction *between* the interviews is what speaks volumes about your personality. Show interest in everything everyone has to say. Throughout the day you will encounter faculty, residents, office administrative staff, nursing staff, hospital staff, and medical students. They are all a part of your future at this institution, and everyone you meet has a say (either directly or indirectly) in your ranking order. Treat them all accordingly.

Keep you cell phone off for the entire day. This should be self-explanatory. Your number one priority today is showing this department that you belong here. Respect their time and efforts with your undivided attention.

"You will not gel with every single person you interview with. That is ok. Don't let this become an awkward silence. Have an interesting story, be polite and personable. You will most likely see the again."

- PK, Physical Medicine and Rehabilitation

What programs are looking for:

What traits are most important to a program director? What exactly are they looking for? Is there anyone with some insight into the mystery that is the Match? If only I could read the minds of the illuminati that control residency admissions...

Unknown to many residency applicants, the answers to the above questions are written in plain English and accompanied by beautiful bar graphs. Recall the previously mentioned *NRMP Program Director Survey* that is freely available online as a PDF. Conveniently for you, it is organized by specialty, and will tell you verbatim what program directors valued in last year's match.

Recall Rule #3: Do Your Homework. Familiarize yourself with the data in this document specific to your specialty of choice.

From the most recent 2014 data (and as was mentioned in the introduction), while USMLE scores are the number one determining factor of who gets an interview invitation, they fall to number *five* when deciding who to rank in the Match.

You'll want to do a bit of a deep dive into the information and figure out where your speciality generally places value. Do Dermatology program directors generally care more about my personal statement or my AOA membership? Do Pediatric program directors generally look for someone more interested in research or someone with a perceived commitment to the specialty? Numbers don't lie. Find out what the program director sitting across from you is looking for in a resident.

Use this knowledge to your advantage and tailor your answers and behavior to demonstrate your strengths in these targeted areas or bring up highlights of your application packet throughout the day.

A more general and perhaps more honest answer to what programs are really looking for is divided between the residents and the faculty.

Residents have short-term goals and are thinking about people they will work with over the next one to six years. Overall, residents want to find someone they will get along with, and can work long hours beside. Ideally a new resident will be someone they can work with, socialize with, and who is generally just a good person. At the very least they want to weed out those who would throw them under the bus to better their careers. Competition is rampant in medicine, and that includes vying for top fellowships and top jobs. One toxic resident with gunner ambitions, slacker tendencies, or poor communication skills can create years of petty catfights and scheduling nightmares for their peers to have to deal with.

Faculty have long-term goals, are more forward thinking, and look at applicants through a wider lens. They consider resident training in the scope of overall departmental and specialty field success. The faculty are looking for someone who has the knowledge and confidence to take care of patients, but enough humility and curiosity to learn new techniques and procedures. They want intelligent, hard workers who have demonstrated the ability to pass licensing tests. Furthermore, they want residents who will make the department look good at both a local and

49

national level. Good communication and strong people skills mean smooth interactions between specialties, good rapport with consultant teams, and clear communication when checking out patients in the middle of the night. Residents with the ability and drive to publish research in journals and present at conferences help the program achieve and maintain a strong reputation, as well as help recruit strong resident classes for years to come. Faculty will also have personal goals involving resident recruitment and training, as departments often use resident education duties as a metric for promotion and tenure.

No matter their rank, your interviewers are tasked with finding out enough supplemental information about you in 15-30 minutes to make a decision about your fit with their program. Programs that spend any time formally training interviewers have them focus on multiple things: remaining neutral in conversations, reading and displaying appropriate body language, and assessing applicant answers on both superficial and profound levels. Typically, they will be taking notes during the interview on a standardized feedback form that will be used when creating the rank order list. Applicant traits listed on these evaluation forms include (but are not limited to): motivation to the specific specialty, professionalism, leadership, resilience, and communication skills. Often these have a scale of one to five or one to ten and are used to translate a subjective conversation into a rough objective "score."

Each of these specific evaluation sheets differ from program to program, and there is no way to "hack" the system. Following the advice laid out in this book, however, will absolutely help you leverage the questions, answers, body language, and overall demeanor you display to score highly in any category on any form - capped off with glowing commentary.

What are the different types of interviews?

The actual interviews themselves can fall into broad categories like individual, group, traditional, and blinded. Each residency program and program director is unique, will have their own style, and can even shift styles mid-season. As such, it is important to be prepared for multiple variables in this setting. Here are some examples of the most common interview types:

Traditional: This is a one-on-one interview between one single interviewer and one single applicant during which the interviewer has access to all subjective and objective data (USMLE scores, CV, medical school transcript, personal statement, letters of recommendation, and GPA). Interviewers often skim the material before the interview to pull questions from, and will often reference line items during your time together for you to clarify or elaborate on.

Blinded: Blinded interviews are also usually between one interviewer and one applicant, except that the interviewer has *not* been given certain information. All objective data is omitted (USMLE scores, medical school name, and grades) and interviewers have only subjective information (personal statement and letters of recommendation) to review. This technique is used to help tease out the best candidates while eliminating bias towards higher scores or specific school names.

Panel: As the name implies, panel interviews are usually conducted between a panel of interviewers and one applicant. While this is possibly the most intimidating interview format, it provides a perfect opportunity for you to get multiple viewpoints of the department as a whole. In addition, panel interviews are the most psychologically nuanced. On a panel of interviewers with varying levels of interviewing expertise, it is possible for residents or even junior faculty to try and impress more senior faculty members or department leadership with "good" questions. To be successful, remain calm and address each question as you would in a one-on-one interview. Try and connect with one or two individuals on a deeper level instead of aiming to please all members of the panel equally.

Group: Group interviews create a more dynamic environment involving one or more interviewers with a small group of three to five applicants. Designed to see how well you interact in group settings, there are many factors at play in these interviews. To shine, you need demonstrate good listening skills and respect for the voice and opinion of others. On the surface these seem biased against introverted personalities, but that is not the case, and far from the goal in these scenarios. Recall Rule #5: Be yourself.

Trust me, a department full of extroverted personalities would be a catastrophe. If you are naturally introverted, interact as you would anywhere else, making a point to be involved as an active listener. Think of the difference between coming across as "eager to learn" and crossing the line to "obnoxious gunner." The same principal applies to an "introspective introvert" crossing the line to "antisocial and disinterested." Program directors want a good mix of both of the former, and neither of the latter.

"If someone is acting obnoxious in a group, disassociate yourself from them immediately. You do not want to be associated with that person during rank list meetings. Residents talk."

-RJ, *Internal Medicine*

Multiple Mini Interview (MMI): The MMI was first introduced in Canada approximately ten years ago, and since then has been gaining popularity in US universities. Much like the USMLE Step 2 Clinical Skills exam, an MMI is set up as a series of short "speed-dating" style questions. Five to ten interviewers ask you only one question each as you rotate from room to room. Questions have been designed to test communication skills, critical thinking, and social intelligence, and your exposure to each interviewer will usually only be 5 to 10 minutes.

Video: Also growing in popularity is the video interview. Using software like Skype, programs can drastically cut down on the amount of time and money applicants spend on travel. A handful of departments currently offer applicants the option of a video interview, and I suspect many more will soon follow suit. Similar to an actual interview day, applicants can interact with faculty, chat with residents, and take virtual tours of hospitals. In April of 2016, the Loma Linda Anesthesiology department published a paper showing that their acceptance rate was the same for applicants who chose face-to-face interviews and applicants who chose web-based interviews.

Telephone: Telephone interviews are usually only reserved for IMGs, but still serve their purposes in limited arenas. Sometimes they are used simply as a test of English comprehension when trying to fill last minute spots in the SOAP. Rarely performed, they are not ideal for either the applicant or the program, and both parties can walk away without a good "feel" for each other. If this is your only option, however, treat it as you would an in-person interview, and every other piece of advice in this book applies.

Who is interviewing you?

As alluded to earlier, you will be interviewed by two levels of interviewers, residents and faculty. Within those two groups, however, experience specific to interviewing resident applicants varies widely. While a program director usually has a polished approach and can tease out nuanced replies, junior faculty not familiar with the process may have a difficult time coming up with questions that allow you to demonstrate your abilities. For example, fifteen minutes of asking yes or no questions about a research paper you contributed to in college is not a good use of time.

If you followed Rule #3 and did your homework, you will at least have a general idea about your interviewer's level of experience before walking in. In addition, you will know their personal and professional interests and be prepared to talk about both.

It is safe to assume that faculty members are comfortable using interview time efficiently, and will have specific questions they like to base their opinions on. Most of the time, however, residents do not receive any formal training on which questions to ask, how to formulate follow up questions, or how to tease out personality traits from responses. Some resident interviews could double as awkward first dates. This is incredibly dangerous, not only because their line of questioning may not be able to get a thorough, accurate assessment of you, but because they have a HUGE say in your ranking.

How do you use this to your advantage? You impress experienced interviewers with your level of preparation, as well as your ability to integrate all of the knowledge you have assimilated by doing your homework. Clear, crisp communication skills and the ability to demonstrate leadership and critical thinking will be evident in your answers.

For inexperienced questioners that fall into a habit of asking closed ended questions that do not allow for much elaboration, know when to interject some of your key selling points. While some conversation is okay to help build rapport, practice redirecting back to your goal of working alongside them in the future. This facetime comes at a premium, and you need to make sure you put your best foot forward for all interviewers.

What types of questions to expect:

There are many "lists" of practice questions you can and should study from. This will not be one of them. Instead, I will break down the types of questions you will be asked, identify the meaning behind them, and highlight what interviewers are looking for in an answer.

Ideally, answers should be well-thought-out and polished while maintaining a candid and conversational tone to avoid sounding stilted or rehearsed. Make sure to play to your strengths and find ways to elaborate on your most positive attributes with all interviewers, tweaking them slightly each time to fit the specific needs of each program. This crucial balance is best achieved with an amount of practice just short of memorization. Do not, however, cross that line.

Be careful rehearsing too many answers to any questions, including the ones that follow, as memorized answers will come across as inauthentic. The correct words said in an incorrect tone will always backfire. Programs want to hear honest, reflective, and thoughtful replies that are unique to each individual. Ron Fry, author of *101 Great Answers to Interview Questions*, eloquently describes a perfect answer as "a unique blend of abilities, skills, and personal qualities - one shaped by your own personal and professional history."

Greeting and small talk:

- *Hello, nice to meet you*
- *How was your trip?*
- *How was dinner last night?*
- *Morning treating you well?*

While these are not considered "formal" interview questions, they are indeed part of your interview.

What are they really asking?

These superficial icebreakers get the conversation flowing. There is no hidden agenda. Rather, this is your chance to make a great first impression.

What do they want to hear?

Confident, clear, positive answers delivered with a smile on your face. If at all possible, be the first to speak. Extend your hand for a firm handshake. Keep a conversational cadence to your answers, and interject a bit of humor if appropriate.

"Dinner was excellent - I think I'm still full!"

"The trip went well, thanks for asking. I was expecting more of a crowd, but have never seen Laguardia that empty."

How you interact with an individual during this quick exchange often dictates the pace of the interview that follows.

Categories of Questions

Questions about you:

- *Tell me a little bit about yourself.*
- *Who would you say "you" are?*
- *How would your friends describe you?*
- *How would your professors describe you?*
- *How do you spend your free time?*

You should absolutely expect these types of questions, and you should be prepared to talk about your unique skills and benefits.

What are they really asking?

There are a few things hidden between the lines of these types of questions. How you perceive yourself, what your passions outside of medicine, and your maturity level can all come through in your replies.

What do they want to hear?

Questions about you answered by you should theoretically be the most authentic and unique portion of the discussion. Deliver a good answer and you are seen as honest, reflective, and trustworthy. Deliver a canned answer you think they want to hear and you will come off as a used car salesman. In addition to maintaining authenticity, make a conscious effort to brag about yourself. High achievers (that includes even low-achieving medical students) are notorious for a stereotypical self-deprecating humor, or a kind of modesty when discussing outstanding test results. There is a time and place for modesty, and it is not when you are trying to stand out among equals. Fight the urge to cheapen your hard work and success.

You are not alone if talking positively about yourself seems a little off-putting to you. In her book, *Brag! The Art of Tooting Your Own Horn Without Blowing It*, author Peggy Klaus explores this uncomfortable feeling in depth. Humility is a virtue with an almost spiritual foundation that is taught from childhood worldwide. Remaining quiet on interview day or downplaying your achievements will not convey passion for your chosen field. Klaus encapsulates a good balance in her definition of "bragging" - *"talking about your best self (interests, ideas and accomplishments) with pride and passion in a conversational manner intended to excite admiration, interest and wonder, without pretense or overstatement – in other words, without being obnoxious."* Throughout this process, you are both the product and the salesperson. No one else is here on your behalf, and you need to step up to the plate.

Specifically, interviewers want to hear a quick "elevator pitch" about what makes you unique, and what would make you the best fit for the team. I recommend combining biographical elements with details about your passion for the field, and specific passions outside of medicine.

Passion outside of medicine may seem counterintuitive, but it speaks volumes about your resilience. Medicine is a difficult field, especially during the long hours of residency training. It is important that you have a stress outlet to recharge the batteries and prevent burnout. You will get bonus points for hobbies that have goals (i.e. running a marathon, climbing a mountain, writing a book) and for activities that involve social volunteer work. Examples:

My closest friends would describe me as a good listener, loyal companion, and an amateur foodie. I found my passion for primary care working in the student run clinic every Saturday, and a close second passion traveling around Texas looking for the perfect queso.

Another possibility:

I have thought long and hard about three things that describe myself on the interview trail, and my answer changes every so often. Because of those changes, I learned that I am more flexible than I ever thought possible, and I can adapt to most situations. If I had to pick another two words, I like persistent and sincere.

Or:

When not studying, I love to spend as much time as possible hiking. I was fortunate enough to grow up around Glacier National Park and find a lot of peace in the outdoors. My certification in Advanced Wilderness Life Support allows me to combine my personal and professional passions. After completing your Emergency Medicine residency I would like to eventually practice in an area that would allow plenty of access to alpine hiking trails.

Questions about your goals:

- *Why do you want to be an Emergency Physician?*
- *What makes St. John's the right fit for you?*
- *Where do you see yourself in five years?*
- *What does the ideal residency look like to you?*
- *What are your post graduation plans?*

What are they really asking?

Questions about your goals are designed to see if your future plans align with what the program can provide. An interviewer can determine if your ambition makes you a good fit for the program, and can identify specific faculty or resources to help you to decide if the program is right for you.

If you want to be an academic clinician, a university setting would be better for you than a community-based program; let an interviewer know you considered this. The opposite is true if you want to practice as a "jack-of-all-trades" primary care physician, and you should highlight this for community-based programs. If you see yourself as a clinician and researcher in the future, mention this to your interviewer, and they can help direct you to departmental resources that will help you make decisions on your rank order list.

What do they want to hear?

Enthusiastic, forward-thinking answers are the best. These can include your previous contributions to the field as examples of how dedicated you are to the profession. Good example answers to these types of questions include:

The faculty focus on Integrative Medicine here at St. John's aligns perfectly with my future plans to include acupuncture in my future practice. I would like to join a small group practice and offer a combination of general primary care, counseling, and integrative medicine options.

Or:

Ideally, I see myself graduating from your anesthesia program, completing a Pain Management fellowship, and then practicing at a major medical center. Five years from now, I would probably be contributing to the body of research in palliative cancer care, an area I have already started to focus on with my research.

Or:

My happiest moments in medical school were in an operating room. I was energized by the hands-on procedures, the quick problem solving, and the ability to produce tangible results. The long hours, 4 AM bandage checks, and tired arms from retracting were more than worth it. I don't know yet if I would choose a fellowship or subspecialty, but I do know I want to get the foundation of my graduate medical education in your general surgery program.

Questions about your chosen profession:

- *Which personality traits do you have that will make you a successful surgeon?*
- *Who inspired your interest in Urology?*
- *Where do you see the field of ENT in 10 years?*

Specialty-specific questions are guaranteed. Interviewers want to know that you have given your decision to be a dermatologist, radiologist, plastic surgeon, or any other kind of physician a good amount of thought.

What are they really asking?

Interviewers want to know that you know what you are getting into at a profound level. Show them that you understand the ins and outs of the profession, and the daily life of residency. Plastic surgery is not all cosmetic procedures, Radiology is not all moonlighting remotely from a yacht in the Baltic sea, and

Emergency Medicine is nothing like what we see on television. They want to make sure you thought seriously and deeply about your profession of choice, and that it is something that you want to wake up every day for.

What do they want to hear?

Good answers will be reflective and forward thinking about specific aspects of the specialty. Comment on what these doctors do on a day-to-day basis to make a living, not the romanticized version. Realities of the medical field include the smell of C. difficile, early morning bandage changes, rectal disimpactions, pimp questions, dealing with death, miscarriages...you know, the hard stuff. What are the rewarding aspects of your chosen specialty that outweigh these negative aspects? Good replies reflect on the profession as a whole and comment on the risks and benefits. One possible example:

On the first day of my neurosurgery elective, I thought it was not really for me. My attending that month was a God in the hospital with hundreds of publications and multiple patents, and I was lucky to even be on the team. Our first case was a traumatic brain injury, and I watched him save a child's life in the OR, and then have to tell her family that she would be forever quadriplegic. The thrill of watching incredible technical skill followed by a somber patient interaction was an absolute roller coaster for me as a student. I was surprised to see how grateful the family was, though, and it helped me reconnect with the reasons I went into medicine in the first place. I saw honesty, empathy, and sincerity in their discussion.

As the rotation progressed, I saw myself drawn to the complexity of skull-based procedures, and I was even able to apply my engineering background by helping a team modify a new aneurysm clip. The patient interactions seemed to come naturally to me, and after that first day, I saw that my mentors were delivering far more good news than bad. Overall, I found myself drawn to the clinical details, the research scope, and the ability to help patients when they need it most. I am certain that neurosurgery is a field I will continue to be passionate about.

Questions about the geographic region:

- *What ties do you have in Boston?*
- *Have you ever been to Denver before?*
- *What is different about Internal Medicine here than at your home institution?*

What are they really asking?

Do you have a good support system in place while you train here, and will you adjust well? In addition, after we spend lots of time and money training you, are you likely to remain in the area and give back to our hospital / community / state?

What do they want to hear?

Residency is an extremely difficult time. Interviewers want to hear that you have friends and family nearby to serve as stress outlets, act as last-minute babysitters, or just to do laundry or cook a home-cooked meal. Make it clear that you will have no problem adjusting to life in this new location.

Residency also serves as another "beginning" in your life as far as career prospects go. New graduates frequently stay on as faculty or end up in practice near their training locations. Everyone knows California is beautiful, and that Denver is near world-class skiing. Those reasons alone are not enough to convince programs you are the best fit for them. Give thoughtful, meaningful answers as to why this specific location is where you want to spend the next few years of your life. One such example:

I don't have any family in Boston, but I did live here for five years when I was younger. I have always wanted to come back, and residency seems like the perfect opportunity. My wife is also originally from New England, and she is very excited about moving back up north.

Or:

My passion is cochlear implants, and as you can see in my application it is a subject I spent the last 3 years researching. I was fortunate enough to meet Dr. Deegan at a conference last year, and after speaking with him for only a short while, I knew that he was a world-class mentor. The chance to train under him is the reason I would choose this program over all others.

Questions about your behavior:

- *Tell me about a stressful patient encounter you had in medical school and how you handled it.*

- *Tell me about at time you disagreed with an attending physician and how you handled the situation.*

- *Tell me about a time you had to build a working relationship with someone you didn't like and what the outcome was.*

- *Tell me about the last time you failed at something.*

"Behavioral" questions ask you to reflect on your previous actions and intentions in order to demonstrate aspects of your personality.

What are they really asking?

The concept here is that past performance dictates future performance. Questions in this area are meant to tease out applicants who are open to personal growth, and who are able to turn difficult situations into positive and tangible lessons.

What do they want to hear?

Interviewers want to know that you are flexible, adaptable, work well in teams, and learn from your mistakes. Ideally, answers to these questions demonstrate your ability to respond to feedback, grow personally, and ultimately develop good leadership skills. Good examples to these types of questions include:

I once had a rotation with a notoriously malicious surgical attending and was dreading our time together. He had a reputation for failing many students for seemingly trivial things, and I knew I needed at least a "high pass" to remain competitive come match day. At the beginning of the rotation, I let the residents on my team know that I was interested in a surgical residency, and asked what I should specifically accomplish and what specifically to avoid. I arrived early every day, stayed late without complaints, knew all of my patients inside and out, studied each operation in detail before setting foot in the OR, and focused on the nuances he was nitpicky on during rounds - specifically knowing the most recent potassium levels, 24-hour surgical drain output, and never rounding with my hands in my pockets. Halfway through the rotation, I asked him personally for feedback on my performance and advice on areas for improvement. He was a man of few words, but seemed at least satisfied with my performance on the team, and I was able to fine-tune a bit of my outside reading and answer more questions in the OR based on his feedback. Not only was I able to achieve the "High Pass" I wanted in surgery, but I learned a lot about staying positive in negative situations, and soliciting feedback early.

Questions about your previous patient cases:

- *What was the most interesting surgical procedure you scrubbed on and why?*
- *Tell me about your most memorable patient experience.*

I recommend knowing at least three patient cases that you have seen. By "knowing" I mean knowing in great detail, similar to presenting to an attending on morning rounds, and being able to discuss lessons learned, actions taken, successes and failures.

What are they really asking?

Medicine is patient care. Even in the dark room of radiology or through the microscopes in a pathology lab, you are fundamentally involved in patient care. Being able to recall and reflect on specific patient cases is necessary for continuing medical education, morbidity and mortality conferences, and publication of case reports. Interviewers want to make sure that this ability is already in your skill set.

What do they want to hear?

There is no need to "wow" an interviewer with medical mysteries here; after all, you will have seen only a fraction of the patients that your interviewer has seen. Simply stick with cases you were personally involved in, and that you found interesting. Consider encounters where you connected with a patient or connected well with their families. Think of cases that you were involved in that required extensive problem solving, or specific instances when you contributed to the team. Use this opportunity to incorporate your critical and clinical thinking skills with personality traits into a cohesive answer. Again, you don't have to have a heroic, "student saves the day" story, but demonstrate sound critical and clinical thought. An example:

I learned a great deal about truly listening to patients in our student-run clinic. One of the more challenging patients well known to the clinic had

CHF with a long list of comorbidities. We couldn't figure out why she had so many hospital admissions for her uncontrolled edema and tried for months to titrate the perfect diuretic dosing regimen. After weeks of reading Up To Date, and consulting nephrology fellows, I had a chance to sit down and talk with her. It turns out she never once took a single Lasix tab prescribed to her. After all of the renal equations and medication interactions we were considering in our heads, no one thought to address the simple act of taking the pills with the patient. Her family believed that "Lasix" was a bad word and the sole factor that ruined both of their parent's kidneys - a belief that she was absolutely unwilling to change. We never could convince her to take Lasix, but were able to change her to another loop diuretic and get her fluid levels under control. From that encounter on, I have made it a point to sit and listen to the health beliefs of each and every patient.

Questions based on ACGME Core Competencies:

- *What does professionalism mean to you?*
- *Describe a difficult patient case you were involved in.*
- *Tell me about a time you were able to work in an interdisciplinary team successfully.*
- *How familiar are you with evidence-based medicine in decision making?*

As previously mentioned, the ACGME has developed specific "competencies" that you will be evaluated on throughout your residency. Following Rule #3 should have you very familiar with these (patient care, medical knowledge, practice-based learning and improvement, interpersonal and communication skills, professionalism, and systems-based practice), and you should expect questions in this area.

What are they really asking?

Interviewers want to know that you understand what will be expected of you in the next few years. Knowing the expectations of the program and how you will be evaluated in the future will make your transition through graduate medical education much more efficient.

What do they want to hear?

Ideal answers should show understanding of what these core competencies are, and should illustrate your ability to recognize both your role in them and their role in your training. For example:

Professionalism to me means putting the honor and integrity of your profession above everything else - in medicine specifically putting patient goals, needs, and beliefs above our personal goals, needs, and beliefs.

Or:

I once had a patient tell me in my ortho rotation how much he learned from the physical therapist. He said that he knew his surgeon exercised incredible skill for a few hours, and that the nursing staff took care of his every need for a few days, but the exercises that his physical therapist gave him were

71

the thing that he valued the most. Those were the things he took home with him for multiple weeks and gave him tangible results he could see and feel. Hearing how empowered he felt was eye opening, and while I have always valued input from our physical and occupational therapy colleagues, I look forward to working more closely with them during my residency in orthopedic surgery.

Questions about clinical decision making:

- *Are you familiar with the new hypertension guidelines?*

- *Tell me what you know about treatment of COPD exacerbations.*

- *If you are paged to the ICU and find an unresponsive patient, what is your first instinct?*

- *Throw a few mattress sutures for me in this banana.*

While not asked often, some programs occasionally incorporate clinical questions into interviews. In theory, interviewers get an idea about your clinical knowledge from your standardized test scores, so these types of questions are rare.

What are they really asking?

Again, the foundation of residency is patient care, and interviewers need to know that you can apply the knowledge you have learned in medical school. IMGs and candidates with borderline test scores report a higher frequency of clinical questions. In these cases, the questions are likely an attempt for the interviewer to verify sound clinical judgement.

What do they want to hear?

Something close to the right answer. Interviewers will not be nitpicky about medication dosages or ventilator settings, but you should have a good idea of how to approach the common conditions you will see in residency. Don't get flustered, remember your basic medicine, and approach the question as you would on rounds. If you truly don't know, it is alright to admit that you are unclear on the specifics and make your best educated guess.

From what I have read and understand, the Joint National Committee-8 increased the hypertension threshold to 140/90 for most individuals. If a patient had an elevated reading with the proper size cuff on two separate occasions, I would recommend lifestyle changes for three months, and then consider a thiazide diuretic as first-line therapy.

And:

Assuming I had never seen the patient before, I would assess the current vital signs, address the ABCs, and check a finger stick glucose, send arterial blood gases, and maybe set up for an EKG if they were not already on a monitor. If those were unstable, I would initiate either a rapid response or code. If the vitals were stable, I would perform a quick chart review including labs and recent medication administrations and ask the nursing staff about any changes in the last few hours.

Questions about your personality:

- *Tell me a joke.*
- *If you were a plant, what type of plant would you be?*
- *Draw a picture of me riding a spaceship.*

These "wildcard" questions are hard to predict, but may be the most fun type of question an interviewer could ask.

What are they really asking?

These questions are used to get a glimpse of your personality. Handling these questions well takes quick thinking, wit, and the ability to not take yourself too seriously.

What do they want to hear?

More important than the quality of any response is maintaining a calm and collected demeanor. Feel free to laugh at yourself, and don't overthink your answers. Have a politically correct, profanity-free joke at the ready. Show you can think on your feet.

I think I would be a cactus. They like the heat of the Arizona outdoors, seem to be pretty low maintenance, and if television hasn't lied to me they can provide water for people stranded in the desert.

Or:

A 44-year-old man lived with his mother for his entire life without muttering a single word. One day at dinner, his first words ever came out of his mouth: "Will you please pass the salt?" Dumbfounded, his mother picked up the salt, slowly gave it to him, and asked the obvious question, "Why now, after all these years, have you never said anything to me?" He replied, "Well, up until now, everything was fine."

Another easy favorite:

Two large antennas met on a roof. They fell in love and decided to get married. The wedding wasn't much but the reception was great.

How to handle difficult questions:

Relax. There is no perfect applicant. Gaps in your record, a failed USMLE score, a failed rotation, legal action, time off - medical students are humans too. These are a few so called "red flags" that are obvious to interviewers even glancing at an ERAS form, and will be of interest to your future employers.

As there is no denying that these types of things will surface during the interview, some self-reflection beforehand can go a long way. Conducting a reflective self-review of your record can help you identify and acknowledge your own personal "red flags." This way, you can prepare answers for all possible scenarios.

Why so cruel? Did they not look at the good parts? See how well I did on Step 2? They did, but success and praise are easy

75

to handle. What interviewers are really looking for when they bring up these negative aspects of your application is how well you deal with adversity.

The right answer to any of these inquiries is to be transparent. Remember, you still got invited to interview. They liked you enough to want you to explain these few "blips" in an otherwise outstanding record. Take responsibility for your actions and explain how you overcame the challenge and experienced personal growth as a result. Some examples:

Interviewer: "I see you got a high pass in all rotations except for Psychiatry, can you tell me a little more about that?"

Applicant: "As you can see my Psychiatry rotation was early in third year, and I did not realize the importance of asking for feedback throughout my rotation. More specifically, I only heard about certain issues my attending was having with me in a final evaluation. I spoke with my advisor and now solicit feedback early on in every rotation to allow me to meet the goals and objectives of each attending."

Interviewer: "I see here that you failed your first attempt on Step 1, what happened there?"

Applicant: "That was an enormous learning opportunity for me, and a very hard pill to swallow. Looking back on it, I think that I just didn't prepare correctly. The reading I did was not as specific to tested topics, and while the question bank I used was an incredible resource, I did not spend enough time with it. For my second attempt, and for Step 2, I took studying much more seriously and dedicated the appropriate amount of time to it, and as you can see did well. I don't see Step 3 or the Internal Medicine boards being a problem for me in the future, and I already have my study plan in place."

The strength of these applicant replies is that they both take ownership, don't slough responsibility, and don't pass blame. They demonstrate to the interviewer that the applicants have put a system in place to prevent it from happening again, and that it is not a sign of poor future performance.

The ERAS application has a section on "legal action" that may also come up and will indeed be classified as a "tough" question. Underage alcohol possession can be chalked up to being young and stupid. Speeding tickets are a dime a dozen. Some of the things you are required to report are unfortunate and fairly common. As above, take ownership, and make it clear that a lesson was learned and a plan is in place to not allow it again.

Overall, it is important to remember that there are very few specific "wrong" answers to even the most difficult interview questions. There are, however, very wrong patterns of answering questions. Refusing to take responsibility for failures, passing blame for any insufficiencies in your CV, not acknowledging your mistakes, or taking full credit for projects that others are clearly involved in are all red flags. Answers demonstrating humility, honesty, and modesty are preferred.

Four answers to avoid at all cost:

Lying: Lack of a specific experience or lack of a specific skill set may not necessarily cost you a job, but lying about it most certainly will.

Belittling your old institution: "Our pharmacology professors were notoriously bad." "Well, you know what they say about ____." When you talk badly about your old institution, we assume you will do this do this for every organization you ever come in contact with. There is no need to sugar coat things either, but figure out a way to shed a positive light on any experience.

Feeling sorry for yourself: "We didn't deliver any babies the whole month." "We never had the chance to see a Whipple." instead, try *"Unfortunately I was not exposed to that at my institution, but it is something I am definitely looking forward to learning more about."* or *"I am excited about the resources and opportunities here to help me broaden my exposure to more surgical procedures."*

Complaining: Do not complain about anything, whether it be your old professor, traffic, food...anything. Complaining makes you look childish, sounds unprofessional, and is not something interviewers will tolerate.

IMG Pearl - There is a good possibility that you will not understand a question or certain words may be unclear. Have no fear - this happens even to native English speakers. Accents are different, slang terms are different, and often the same word means different things depending on which region of the US you are in.

Even if you trained in an English-speaking UK system, medication names, disease names, and recommendations will differ slightly from US versions. Simply say that you do not quite understand the question, and politely ask your interviewer to restate or rephrase it. A pause while processing your answer is fine as well; there is no penalty for pausing to organize your thoughts.

How to handle illegal questions:

We all hear about "illegal" questions in the eyes of the NRMP. Often these are not malicious, and are mostly designed to keep a level playing field between all applicants and programs. The current NRMP policy explicitly states:

"Program directors shall recognize the negative consequences that can result from questions about age, gender, religion, sexual orientation, and family status, and shall ensure that communication with applicants remains focused on the applicant's goodness of fit within their programs."

Furthermore, US federal law prevents employers from basing hiring decisions on sexual orientation, marital status, religion, race, color, nationality, veteran status, disability, family planning, or children. These rules apply to all jobs, not just residency positions.

"Legal" communication in the eyes of the NRMP also includes questions about where applicants have applied, what specialties they applied to, where they ranked, etc and are covered later in the book.

While technically labeled as "illegal" - some issues surface as a result of questions you may ask. For example, a program director can not ask if you have children, but if you ask multiple questions about childcare, we can assume that you either have a child or are at least thinking of having one. An interviewer can not ask you if you are a religious person, but if you wear clothing specific to one religion, we can assume you follow certain religious practices. The list goes on.

These things come up for a variety of reasons, most of which are benign and just part of the conversation flow. Do not overreact. Remember Rule #2: Know Your Goal. You want a job with these people, but also need to feel comfortable working with them for the next few years. Minor slip ups are to be expected; it's a conversation, not a court of law. If you think the mistake was unintentional, no worries. However, If you think the questions seem inappropriate to you, you need to be concerned. How you proceed is up to you. There is no big red "eject" button, and no red phone for you to pick up. Do your best to emphasize that whatever the answer is, it will not affect your job: Examples:

Interviewer: Looking at your CV you seem to be very involved with your children's school activities? How are you able to keep up with the demands of medical school?

Applicant: "My children are obviously very important to me, and I make time to be a part of their life. Similarly, my career is extremely important to me, and I take the necessary time to excel in school."

Interviewer: As a Muslim myself, I struggle each year when Ramadan rolls around. Would you like us to schedule you for night float during that month?

Applicant: "While I appreciate the consideration, I am pleased with the job I have done thus far balancing my personal and professional life, and I don't anticipate a problem with it in the future."

As you can see, if these issues come up at all, they are often hidden in well-intentioned questions. Curiosity and friendliness can cause people to cross certain lines more often than malice. Whatever your approach, do not respond aggressively and convey the message that your career is a priority.

The real Catch-22 of illegal questioning is that it often involves issues that are important to your decision making. If you want to be close to a specific church, or you want your kids to go to a specific school, you have every right to ask about those things. The rules are put in place to protect YOU from discrimination, not to allow programs to withhold information. You are allowed to ask programs these types of questions; they, however, are not allowed to make hiring decisions based on this information.

Conspiracy theorists among you will ask: "Well, if I ask about temples nearby, they will know I'm Jewish." or "If I ask about day care availability, they will know I have kids." This is true, and if you want to avoid these topics you can. If information listed in this "illegal" space will make all the difference between your happiness and misery over the next three to eight years, however, it may be worth taking that risk and exposing these details.

In the event that a question or line of questioning makes you feel uncomfortable, or clearly crosses the line into "illegal" territory without even the sense that it is inadvertent, it needs to be brought to someone's attention. However, doing this can be tricky. Let's assume a resident says:

"You are not going to get pregnant are you? Man... it is always a nightmare scheduling maternity leave. Last year we had two girls deliver on the same day! The rest of us were pissed that we had to cover for them and never want to go through that again."

I would recommend following the steps above, realize that the resident is an inexperienced interviewer, and deflect answering the question directly, while assuring him that your focus is on your upcoming medical training.

At the end of the day, pull the program coordinator aside and let them know exactly what happened. They may immediately get the program director involved. If neither of these individuals is available at the end of the day, email the program director directly (this is one of the few exceptions where I would recommend this) with the program coordinator cc'ed on the message as soon as you get back to your hotel; do not delay. Leave all contact information, including phone number and email. They WILL call you and will want to know specifically what happened as this is a flagrant violation and will reflect poorly on the program.

In the context of this example, I would NOT go directly to the NRMP / ACGME. If there is one isolated person or problem, the program will deal with it internally. With enough of this type of feedback, problem residents can be fired, as their behavior reflects poorly on the entire program. Rarely do the opinions and voices of the few reflect those of the whole, and I recommend giving programs a chance to make things right without involving licensing boards. ACGME or NRMP punishments can affect dozens of people and cost tens of thousands of literal dollars in man hours and sensitivity training for the actions of one bad apple.

If, however, this same line of commentary was delivered by the program director, then absolutely report it to the NRMP and ACGME. They are on your side, and want residents to be trained in a fair environment. The training program deserves a better leader, or at least one who follows federal law.

That being said, if it is a real debacle, you have every right to report them to an even higher authority, the Federal Equal Employment Opportunity Commission. Hopefully none of you have to take it that far.

Suspected violations must be sent in writing to:

National Resident Matching Program

2121 K Street, N.W.

Washington, D.C. 20037

Fax: 202-354-4586

E-mail: investigations@nrmp.org

What questions you should ask:

One of the most important interactions on interview day will be your opportunity to "turn the tables" and ask your interviewer questions. If you have followed Rule #3 and done your homework, you should have a long list ready to go. Much like the earlier breakdown of types of interview questions you will be asked, I think it is important to think of the types of questions you should ask departments in a similar manner.

The questions you should ask your interviewers will be very specific to you, your professional goals, and your personal lifestyle. There is no definitive list of things you "must" ask as every applicant is different. A single female MD/PhD applicant looking to enter fellowship after residency and ultimately practice in a large academic center has very different goals and expectations than a married father of three looking to join a private group practice immediately after residency. Good sources of question lists include the AAMC, your dean's office, and other online resources, but do not read them off like a laundry list to your interviewer. Reflect on what is important to you personally and professionally, and build your line of questioning around a few core values. It is perfectly acceptable to have these questions written down in your notepad, and to take short notes during the replies.

The following explanations of each area of questioning mirror those seen on the AAMC's *Organization of Resident Representatives* (available for free online, link in references). I think they do a good job capturing the most important information.

Ask questions about the *quality of education.* Residency is, after all, primarily educational. It is important to see exactly how much emphasis is placed on making education of residents a priority. The department as a whole has many other branches, including research, medical student education, and patient care, and department chairs can allocate resources to any one of these branches. Residents can sometimes feel that they are on the wrong end of this hospital machine and end up buried in "scut" work, slaving along in the middle of the night so that attendings can sleep in and make their tee time on Saturday. "Protected" education time means dedicated time set aside exclusively for education, not patient care, research, or any other resident training. Good training programs will make sure that there is structure built around formal education in things like morning report, journal club, morbidity and mortality conferences, etc. In addition, large teaching hospitals and subspecialties have teams that include overzealous medical students gunning for a good LOR as well as fellows who seem to take "all the good cases" while residents can be lost in the mix during their training wound checks and paperwork in clinic out of the OR. Make sure to get a good idea of how this department values resident-specific education.

85

Is there a formal, protected didactic curriculum for residents, and what is its structure?

What platforms exist for resident education? (lectures, journal clubs, board review)

Are there any required rotations that take place outside of the city?

Are there any opportunities to do away rotations?

Is there a formal mentoring program for new residents?

Ask questions about *any available research opportunities*. If you are looking to stay in academic medicine, or hoping to apply to a fellowship position after residency, you will need research experience on your CV. These questions will let you know how the program values research, as well as what resources are in place. "Protected" research time means dedicated time set aside exclusively for research - not patient care, education, or any other resident training. Departments that present at conferences regularly or have prolific published faculty often have some degree of dedicated time, formal training on how to prepare manuscripts or posters, and even graphic design departments to help submit published work.

Conversely, if your ultimate goal is to be a rural primary care physician, research will not be high on your priority list. Some research is usually required during all residency training regardless of specialty, but you can use answers to these questions to shift your focus away from research-heavy programs and focus on a different skill set for life outside of academic medicine.

Are research opportunities provided to residents?

Is resident research required?

Is there "protected" time for research?

Is attendance at regional and national conferences encouraged? Is funding available?

Ask questions about *student teaching responsibilities*. Much like the residents you have been learning from on the wards, once you cross over into residency you too will be thrown into the proverbial deep end. Over time, you will gain the practical experience needed to pass a few pearls of wisdom to eager medical students, but what exactly will your responsibilities be and will you be formally trained on how to facilitate student learning? Most departments will carve out some didactic learning on how to best interact with medical students as well as how to provide feedback and formally evaluate student performance. Even though you will likely only be asked to provide written feedback and evaluation as a senior-level resident, it is important to ask now (before entering the program) to ensure your continued growth as a physician educator. This is especially true if you see yourself practicing in an academic institution after graduation.

What teaching responsibilities for medical students are expected of residents?

Is there any formal training for residents on how to teach students?

Is there any formal training for residents on how to give feedback?

Ask questions about *resident clinical duties*. The meat of your residency experience will involve clinical duties and patient care. This hands-on learning is what gives you the tools and experiences that transform you from a book-smart medical student into an artful clinician. Patient load, case numbers, procedure types, patient population, and your personal involvement in daily patient care all have a direct influence on your skill set at graduation. It is important to find out what your responsibilities will be at each level of residency, where you are utilized as part of the medical team, and how your clinical skills set builds throughout your training.

It is also important to not have unrealistic expectations, as you will not get to scrub on every lung transplant the department performs as a PGY-1. Making sure the program has a stable transplant surgical service with large numbers, though, should mean that you get enough exposure to those cases in your senior years.

What is the general call schedule?

What provisions are made for backup call or sick call coverage?

What type of structure for resident supervision is in place?

How does resident autonomy change as we progress through the program?

Does the general volume of clinical work support a balance between service and education?

Do your residents express that they see enough _____ cases?

Ask questions about *evaluation of resident performance.* Throughout your residency, you will be evaluated according to the ACGME's *Six Core Competencies.* Again, these are: patient care, medical knowledge, practice-based learning and improvement, systems-based practice, professionalism, and interpersonal skills and communication. Know what each of those mean, and know how to demonstrate them to your attendings.

Your promotion from year to year will require evaluation and feedback sessions with multiple faculty advisors using these core competencies as milestones. Departments conduct these evaluations in different ways, and it is important to know how a particular department conducts them and how often you will receive feedback on your performance. In addition, frequent and practical feedback can help you continue to build your CV and focus your efforts when applying to fellowships or jobs in the field. Good programs will have a dedicated one-on-one face-to-face feedback session with a faculty advisor or mentor to help you achieve your future goals.

Objective evaluations in the form of standardized in-training exams are also a tool utilized in most residencies. This is the time to find out what tests the program uses, what resources are available to you to prepare, and what the outcomes mean for your overall evaluation.

How often are residents evaluated?

What is the structure of the evaluation? (forms, face to face)
What other forms of feedback does the resident receive?

Ask questions about *program performance.* The ACGME conducts accreditation hearings of each and every residency program to grant accreditation for zero to ten years. Accreditation is often seen as a "background" issue that is taken for granted, as many hospitals have stellar reputations and are assumed to have the highest level of accreditation. This could not be further from the truth.

Meeting the educational standards set by the ACGME is no easy task, and preparing for a formal review requires months of preparation. Despite the subjective clout some big name hospitals carry, they are not always the best training environments as measured by these rigorous standards. Although they are now well within compliance, programs at both Yale (General Surgery) and Johns Hopkins (Internal Medicine) were famously stripped of their accreditations in the early 2000's for repeatedly violating duty hour restrictions.

While it does not necessarily affect your career prospects if you come from a program who received only a 3-year accreditation as opposed to a 10-year, it does reflect poorly coming from a program who has repeated violations. Most data of this type can be found online, but much like any "red flags" on your personal record, residency programs can have reasonable explanations for their own mistakes and failings. Do not hesitate to ask about them in a curious, non-confrontational manner, as they will absolutely affect your future. Good programs will be transparent about these issues, and will be able to provide explanations of any concerning figures.

What is the status of the program's accreditation?

When is the next RRC review?

Are there any plans for changing program size or structure?

What is the status of the last ACGME review?

What percentage of residents complete the program?

What percentage of your graduates pass the specialty boards on their first attempt?

Where do your graduates go? (fellowship / academics / private practice)

Ask questions about *general employment issues.* This is, after all, a job. You will need to have a basic understanding of work hour restrictions, sick leave, benefits, and health insurance. Many of these are standardized across all programs, and can be found online. Residents can be asked about details such as parking, meal plans, moonlighting, and discretionary funds if you are unable to find this information online. Often, the residents are closer to these issues and can tell you of their own personal experiences.

What are the basic benefits?

Is parking a concern for residents at your program?

Are meals paid for when on call?

Is there reimbursement for educational supplies and books?
Are moonlighting opportunities available?
Is there a House Officers Association at the hospital?

Ask *personal questions* of the residents. Much like the environment at the resident dinner, a certain air exists in resident interviews that is a bit more relaxed. In addition, residents are actually living residency, and they will have answers to some specific questions that faculty could never begin to answer. Competition between specialties for cases, nursing attitudes towards specific specialties, cooperation between current residents, and many other day-to-day issues are all dealt with on the "front lines" by working residents, not their supervisors. This is your chance to ask them. Some of the AAMC's examples will be more appropriate conversation for dinner, some for a more focused interview environment:

Would you consider the same program if applying again?
Is there an appropriate balance between service obligations and educational program?
Is there enough ancillary support to minimize "scut work"?
What has changed since you came to the program?
How accessible are the faculty members?
Do the residents get along with one another?
How do your residents get along with those in other programs?
In what activities are you involved outside of the program?

How does your spouse like the city/area?

Where do most of the residents live?

What are some favorite rotations or favorite elective opportunities?

How is the precepting in clinic?

What is the average daily OR caseload / clinic patients / hospital patients?

Do you feel safe in the community?

How do you find the cost of living?

Do you know of any employment opportunities for a spouse?

Any good schools or daycare for children?

Body Language:

As is any other interaction between two human beings, a residency interview is ripe with psychological nuance. By some measures, how you carry yourself can be more important that what you say. Delivering appropriate body language as well as the ability to interpret the body language of your interviewer will serve you well during interview day. Don't overreach and psychoanalyze your hosts, just be aware of the psychological elements at play when two people meet each other for the first time, and help tip the scales in your favor.

Dr. Albert Mehrabian, a leading Psychology professor at UCLA, has published studies indicating that body language accounts for over 50% of the receiver's understanding, tone of voice accounts for almost 40% and the actual words account for *only* 7% of the receiver's understanding of a message. Think of the last time you heard, "It was not what you said, but the way you said it" and you will understand. Countless books have been written on body language alone, from the poker tells of winning players to successful posturing during negotiation. You want to project confidence without arrogance. Following a few items on this short list will help solidify a good first impression on interview day.

Have a strong entrance: Walk into rooms with your head up and shoulders back, smile, make eye contact, and offer a firm handshake when meeting each new person. If possible, be the first to speak and introduce yourself.

Wait confidently: Sit up straight with your head up and shoulders back, not hunched over and head down. This will make you feel (and appear) more confident.

Act calm, cool, and collected: Do not frantically search for anything in your car, folio, or pockets. Smooth, slow movements convey a greater sense of control.

Actively listen: Lean slightly forward when speaking or listening, with your head tilted slightly to either side. Leaning back in a chair or throwing your arm over the back of another is too comfortable, coming across as borderline arrogant. You can nod your head slightly while the interviewer is talking to imply listening.

Mirroring: Subtly change your voice cadence and demeanor to match that of your interviewer. If they have their arms crossed, you can do the same; if they have a soft, smooth, and slow voice, don't answer with loud, rapid, choppy answers

Hand gestures: Keep your hands above desk but below your head you do not to appear to be hiding anything or to be frantic. When walking, keep your hands out of your pockets.

Be enthusiastic: Don't over do it; you don't need to act like you are at Disneyworld. Show your interest by not checking your phone or looking out the window. Give your undivided attention to your hosts.

Smile: A genuine smile indicates happiness, conveys a friendly attitude, and demonstrates interest. Forced smiles, smirks, and tight-lipped smiles on the other hand, can all indicate suspicious attitudes. Watch a few YouTube videos to spot the difference - hint: *orbicularis oculis.*

Eye contact: Eye contact is expected to be regular, but not overly persistent. Calm blinking conveys honesty, dilated pupils and raised eyebrows can convey interest, and answering questions without looking down conveys trust.

The "Second Look":

Program directors shall respect the logistical and financial burden many applicants face in pursuing multiple interactions with programs and shall not require them or imply that second visits are used in determining applicant placement on a rank order list. - NRMP Communication Code of Conduct

Residency programs have an option to invite applicants to return to the hospital for a second visit. These are designed to give applicants a closer look into a "typical day" in the life of a resident, and will likely come up during your interview day.

A program director will say things along the lines of: "If you would like to organize a second look, just contact the program coordinator and we can set something up."

Theoretically, an environment outside of the formal interview sheds new light on program details that may not be covered in a conversational setting, and asking about or accepting the invitation for a second look does imply interest in a program. However, there is no such thing as a "typical day" and it is unreasonable to think that anything you experience in those four to eight hours would make that program look better to you, or make you look better to the program. Program directors know this, and often extend the interview for second looks as a formality.

No formal data exist equating scheduling a second look and moving up a rank order list.

If you had a solid interview performance, and have a strong application, a second look is unnecessary. The financial burden is indeed significant, but more importantly you take an enormous risk by walking into a situation that is more likely to expose weaknesses than strengths. As an interview applicant with strong letters of recommendation, a strong personal statement, and strong interview skills, you leave an outstanding impression on interview day, and leave the program wanting more. Walking into a well-oiled surgical hospital team, or efficient outpatient medical clinic you will be "on the spot" in a very foreign environment. Standing in the wrong place, leaning on the wrong thing, asking the wrong question, getting pimped on rounds, not having the right answers...all of these could count against you.

I would recommend organizing a second look only if you have the means, get invited, and think you had a terrible interview day. Not that you interviewed poorly, mind you, but that somehow external consequences did not give you a good picture of your future employer. Fire alarms constantly going off, evacuating because of a bomb threat, car accident made you three hours late, half of the faculty stuck at an airport coming back from a conference - you get the idea. There is very little you can do to make up for poor people skills or a weak application, but if you really would like to get a better feel for a program, use the second look to your advantage. Otherwise, it is okay to politely decline.

PART THREE:
THE AFTERMATH

"To be interesting, be interested."

- Dale Carnegie

PART THREE: THE AFTERMATH

Back at home, on a treadmill working off the lobster bisque from last week, you start to reflect on your interview day. You nailed it. Smiles, firm handshakes, great jokes, they loved you. Now what?

Or, conversely: Worst. Day. Ever. You didn't mention your upcoming publication, you sneezed on one of them, misspelled "otolaryngology" in your personal statement, and they were staring at your giant pimple the entire time.

However the day went, now begins the delicate dance of communicating with your dream program at a time when strict rules dictate what you can and can't say.

Corporations in a non-medical environment often make hiring and firing decisions within a single business day (a matter of hours). The residency interview process, however, lasts at least 3 months. The challenge is how to stay relevant weeks after the interview day is over.

Despite the general notion among applicants that all communication is bad, communication occurs often and most of the time falls well within the rules set by the NRMP. While the Match is hardly a cutting-edge area of research, there are a handful of papers measuring certain variables pertaining to successful applicants. These published studies show that anywhere from 65%

to 85% of applicants report communicating with programs following their interviews. In one paper, 95% of program directors say they initiate follow-up communication with applicants.

The NRMP Match Code of Conduct reads:

"Program directors shall not solicit or require post-interview communication from applicants, nor shall program directors engage in post-interview communication that is disingenuous for the purpose of influencing applicants' ranking preferences.

Program directors and other interviewers may freely express their interest in a candidate, but they shall not require an applicant to disclose ranking preferences, ranking intentions, or the locations of other programs to which the applicant has applied or may apply."

This lawyer-speak leaves room for interpretation of what exactly *is* allowed, but is very clear on what constitutes violations. Post-interview communication is also a topic that has more peer-reviewed publications than anything else previously discussed in this book. The results may surprise you.

Some programs explicitly follow a "zero-communication" policy following your interview. You will not be contacted by them, and they will not answer any communication from you that is not directly related to program questions or clarification. No thank you cards will be opened. Respect these boundaries, and follow their policies to the letter. If you want to work at this hospital, at least show them that you can follow rules.

For programs that do not specifically state this policy, however, communication channels and the anxiety that accompany them are open in both directions. Applicants interested in outstanding programs feel the need to contact them in order to stay relevant, and programs interested in outstanding candidates feel the need to contact them in the name of recruitment.

In either the situation, be careful about the content and frequency of your communication with programs. Unless an individual resident or faculty member gave you contact information inviting communication, the program coordinator remains your sole contact in this process. He or she will direct your questions to those best suited to answer them. Calling anyone multiple times daily and e-mailing multiple faculty members is inappropriate. Relevant, genuine questions, on the other hand, come across as authentic, and program coordinators are more than happy to get you the answers you need.

A 2014 paper in the *Journal of Graduate Medical Education* found that applicants who did communicate with programs were no more likely to be ranked in the top half of the rank list than those who did not. Furthermore, applicants who stated they were ranking programs "first" or "very highly" were given similar rank order preference to those who did not communicate at all.

In fact, based purely on published data, it seems as though you have nothing to gain by communicating with programs after interviewing, and may expose yourself to misleading statements and even violations. So, if you do choose to engage in these communications, do so at your own risk.

Interpreting Communication Nuances

"You are a fine example of a competitive candidate who would rank extremely high on our list of applicants."

"Your application makes you one of our top choices."

"The faculty and I are highly interested in your research."

As mentioned before, some programs have adopted a "zero-communication" policy and will have no communication with any applicant - from their number one choice to those who do not even make the rank order list. This can be frustrating, but it is following the letter of the law. Do not get discouraged and take their lack of communication as a lack of interest. Rank them where you see appropriate.

On the other side of the spectrum, some programs routinely contact applicants to "express interest," and open a line of communication for future questions. One or two residents who felt a connection with you will reach out via email or phone call with the blessing of the program coordinator. While this in no way should be misinterpreted as a guaranteed spot, it can be an indication that a program is definitely interested. Feel free to direct your questions to this individual.

Per the NRMP guidelines, you are not obligated to communicate with these individuals in any way. Not communicating will not affect your rank order. Programs respect the anxiety surrounding the Match and NRMP guidelines and will not change your place on a rank list if you choose not to communicate with them.

It is perfectly acceptable to remain in contact with programs weeks or months after your interview. In fact, it is a fantastic way to stay relevant and on their minds. Remain professional, keep it short, and ensure it can not be answered on the department web site.

"St. John's is my #1 choice."

"St. Luke's is at the top of my rank list."

"My wife and I are very interested in both programs, and see ourselves as a good fit."

Be authentic in your communication, personalize your messages, and be honest. Don't tell ten programs that you "ranked them number one," and don't make false promises that can not be backed up. If you are not going to "see them at the conference in May," then don't tell them that. Consider these messages as building on the conversation you had during the interview, and an extension of your application.

The same study of the successful Plastic Surgery applicants found that of the 75% who made contact with programs, 50% of those overstated their interest in the program.

The vital understanding of any post-interview communication is that it should not be misinterpreted. I know that it is hard not to read between the lines when this decision is steeped in so much emotion, but no one can guarantee you anything.

The NRMP algorithm determines who goes where. Therefore, a program director or even a chairman can not promise you a spot in the program. The spots are not theirs to give. In the end, there are absolutely no guarantees in this process.

A 2012 study in *Academic Medicine* found that programs used language such as "ranked to match" (34%), "ranked highly" (52%), or "fit well" (76%) when corresponding with applicants. However nearly 20% of the applicants responding to their survey stated that they felt assured by a program that they would match there and did not despite ranking that program first on their list. In addition, an astonishing 94% of program directors polled in a 2000 paper in the *Journal of Family Medicine* felt that the NRMP process placed them in a position of having to be dishonest with applicants in order to match their top choices.

For those of you who do choose to communicate appropriately with your programs following the interview day, you will usually be sending either thank you cards or program-specific questions. In order to make them count, your words need to be crisp, clear, and concise.

Writing the Perfect Thank You Note

The most common form of post-interview communication is the thank you note. For programs that explicitly state that they do not allow them, do not send them. For everyone else, send a *handwritten* thank you card.

Critics will say the practice is outdated.

"I saw twenty people at ten different programs. I don't have that kind of time."

"My merits should stand on their own. I'm happy with my CV and interview."

"None of my friends are writing thank yous. I don't want to seem different. I'll just e-mail."

Perhaps an outdated and dying art, the handwritten thank you card is a physical symbol of appreciation for the time and effort someone took to interview you. It will stand out for the right reasons, and keep your name fresh in the program director's mind.

Conversely, e-mail is a perfectly acceptable way to send an interview follow-up message or specific question. I would maintain that since medicine is a more traditional, conservative discipline, a handwritten thank you is more of a cultural fit. The physicians you are trying to impress did not grow up with email and were writing thank you cards themselves when in your shoes.

Furthermore, consider how many junk messages you get. A program director's inbox is exponentially worse. E-mail is easy to glaze over, and even easier to forget. I recommend reserving the use of e-mail for programs you have only a mild amount of interest in ranking. For your dream program, and especially to a person (of any status) who you had a connection with, take the time to write a card.

When the odds are against you, every little bit helps. With some programs choosing to interview only 1% of total applicants, it makes sense to be the 1% who takes the time to hand write a card in order to stand out.

Still skeptical? If you must compromise, e-mail some individuals who interviewed you (i.e. the residents at dinner, junior faculty members), and mail only a few handwritten cards (to a program director, future research mentor, or anyone you had a strong personal connection with).

The ultimate goal of the art of the thank you note is to express genuine appreciation for the interviewer's time. Any other primary objective will backfire and come across as forced. Secondary aims are to refresh the program's memory of your character qualities, restate your enthusiasm, and express your motivation to be hired. Here are some suggestions:

Be prompt: Write and mail the note within 48 hours after leaving the interview. This allows you time to reflect on what you want to say, but not too long to forget specifics.

Be personable: Mention a specific story, article, or detail that came up during your interview. This helps refresh a unique talking point that will stand apart from the USMLE scores and CV details that are similar among all candidates.

Be concise: Aim for three to five sentences. Long enough to say what you want to say, but short enough to read. Don't ramble.

Brag: Restate your specific interest in your chosen field, and the specific program. Remind them why you are a good fit. Convey the message that you are the right person for the job, the program meets your needs, and you will represent the program well. Restate your value. Fix any mistakes you made, or say something that you didn't get a chance to say.

It goes without saying that the note needs to be free of any errors. You can type it out first to get an automatic spell check if you must lean on technology. Get a friend to proofread, and take your time to make your handwriting legible. Remember, this may be your last bit of communication with the department until the match; you want to leave a lasting and positive impression. Here's an example:

Dr. Green,

Thank you very much for taking the time to interview me. I truly enjoyed my time at St. John's. I wanted to let you know that since we spoke last, I have submitted an abstract to the upcoming American College of Surgeons conference, and will let you know if it gets accepted. After meeting all of the faculty involved with bariatric surgical procedures, I am certain that St. John's would be a perfect place to start my career. Thanks again, and I'm looking forward to trying out that running trail you mentioned!

Myers Hurt

How to Ask Follow-Up Questions

As you interview at multiple programs, questions will inevitably come up that you forgot to ask other programs earlier on the trail. Attention will be drawn to areas of interest you did not consider important until you hear multiple residents tell you "they should have asked." Parking, meal plans, grand rounds presentations - almost everything is important when trying to ascertain the benefits of one program over another. These are perfect examples of appropriate questions to ask via email. Keep the number of questions to a minimum, and do not pester anyone. Again, this is no time to stand out for the wrong reasons.

Strategically speaking, some communication is a good way to keep your name fresh in the minds of decision makers. One to three well-timed questions can demonstrate genuine interest in a program as well as keep your name relevant in rank list meetings. Authenticity is key, and you should not ask anything you can find out online. Obviously, do not ask anything just for the sake of asking.

Recruiting outstanding applicants is in the best interest of programs, and they will often go out of their way to make themselves available to clarify any issues you have. I would go so far as to say that questions are not only expected, but *welcomed* by all program coordinators.

The one off-limit area is your rank order, or any specifics surrounding your place on a rank list. It is extremely inappropriate and a violation of NRMP guidelines to request such information, and this should be avoided at all costs.

Communicating with programs is absolutely not required in order to rank highly. If you have no questions, or can find the answers on your own, don't sweat it.

Final Pearls

"When you come out of the storm, you won't be the same person who walked in. That's what this storm is all about."

- Haruki Murakami, Author

Final Pearls

Sitting down to compile your rank order list after the interview trail, the tables will turn, and you will find yourself choosing between many objectively similar programs with minor differences between each. Objectively, they will look very similar. Same number of years, same educational focus, same pathways of graduates. Each of them well groomed, wearing a nice suit, holding a leather folder with two pens, and looking you in the eye while giving you a metaphorical firm handshake.

Taking it all in, you are left with the most important questions in the entire Match process - the questions to *ask yourself*. Approaching your applications, you may have asked: *Where do I want to apply?* Interview invitations then narrowed that down to a list you filtered with: *Where do I want to interview?* and finally you are left with: *Where do I want to train?*

If you used an smartphone app, you may have a few lines of 1-5 stars reviewing resident morale, confidence in training, cost of living, and proximity to family. Reviewing your notes, you can see things that make each place attractive to train or live. Faculty advisors, friends, and family can also help you weigh factors in your decision.

As this is no easy decision, you will spend hours weighing pros and cons of very similar programs. Specific faculty, geographic region, or minor details will help you differentiate (and determine preference) for one program over another. Most of the time, you can not go wrong. Diabetes is diabetes, a Whipple is a Whipple, and an ICU in Boston is similar to an ICU in San Francisco. You will emerge a competent physician with six-figure employment prospects.

The most important factor is your *happiness*. Can you really be happy here? You will be spending the next few years with these people, and will turn colleagues into either lifelong friends or sworn enemies. Is a big name hospital worth putting up with distant faculty? Is that program you love in Arizona worth moving your family across the country? Are you willing to sacrifice your ego for that one small program you really loved? You will be facing huge life decisions, and you are looking at starting some of the hardest working years of your life.

This really is a "choose with your heart, not with your head" decision.

"Picking a program based on where you want to live and where you will be happy is more important than prestige. These days, you can Google or YouTube almost anything you need to know instantly."

- BT, Plastic Surgery

I will leave you with one final pearl: make sure that you control the elements of your happiness that you can. Those elements are different for each individual and have to be decided for yourself. No blog post or book can give you the answer. Take time to reflect on your personal and professional goals, and choose to rank programs that can most consistently align with them.

Congratulate yourself on completing this rite of passage, and for surviving a whirlwind of travel, first impressions, and selling yourself. Hopefully the time you have invested in this book has left you feeling confident about your prospects, and comfortable with your choices. Come February, set your rank order list, take a deep breath, and wait for Match day! Opening that envelope is a feeling like no other. Good luck doctor!

References

PART ONE

Trademark:
ACGME and RRC are registered trademarks of the Accreditation Council of Medical Colleges.
Airbnb is a registered trademark of Airbnb, Inc.
Capital One and Venture are registered trademarks of Capital One Financial.
Chase and Sapphire Preferred are registered trademarks of JP Morgan Chase & Co.
Couchsurfing is a registered trademark of Couchsurfing International Inc.
ERAS, MyERAS, SOAP, Scramble, and AAMC are registered trademarks of the American Association of Medical Colleges.
Google is a registered trademark of Google Inc.
Interview Broker is a registered trademark of The Tenth Nerve, LLC.
KevinMD is a registered trademark of KevinMD, LLC.
magicJack is a registered trademark of magicJack VocalTek Ltd.
MATCH and NRMP are registered trademarks of the National Resident Matching Program.
MATCH Prism is a registered trademark of the National Resident Matching Program.
New York Times is a registered trademark of The New York Times Company.
Skype is a registered trademark of Skype.
Swap & Snooze is a registered trademark of Swap&Snooze.
Thalamus is a registered trademark of SJ MedConnect Inc.
Tide is a registered trademark of Procter & Gamble.
TripIt is a registered trademark of Concur Technologies, Inc.
Uber is a registered trademark of Uber Technologies Inc.

Fry, Ron, *101 Answers to the Toughest Interview Questions: Sixth Edition.* Career Press, 2012.

Klaus, Peggy. *Brag! The Art of Tooting Your own horn without Blowing it.* Business Plus, 2008

National Resident Matching Program, Data Release and Research Committee: *Results of the 2014 NRMP Program Director Survey.* National Resident Matching Program, Washington, DC; 2014.

National Resident Matching Program, *Charting Outcomes in the Match, 2014.* National Resident Matching Program, Washington, DC; 2014.

National Resident Matching Program, Data Release and Research Committee: *Results of the 2015 NRMP Applicant Survey by Preferred Specialty and Applicant Type.* National Resident Matching Program, Washington, DC; 2015.

PART TWO

Trademark:
Betadine is a registered trademark of the Purdue Frederick Company.
Kleenex is a registered trademark of the Kimberly-Clark Corporation.
Skype is a registered trademark of Skype.
Walt Disney World is a registered trademark of Disney Enterprises, Inc.

Vadi MG et al. *Comparison of web-based and face-to-face interviews for application to an anesthesia training program: a pilot study.* Int J Med Educ. 2016 Apr 3;7:102-8.

PART THREE

Carek PJ et al. *Recruitment behavior and program directors: how ethical are their perspectives about the match process?* Fam Med. 2000 Apr;32(4):258-60.

Don't Forget to Ask: Advice from Residents on What to Ask During the Residency Interview.
https://www.aamc.org/download/77936/data/residencyquestions
.pdf

Dort JM et al. *Applicant characteristics associated with selection for ranking at independent surgery residency programs.* J Surg Educ. 2015 Nov-Dec;72(6):123-9.

Frishman GN et al. *Postinterview communication with residency applicants: a call for clarity!* Am J Obstet Gynecol. 2014 Oct;211(4):344-350.

Iglehart, John. *The Residency Mismatch.* N Engl J Med 2013; 369:297-299 July 25, 2013 DOI: 10.1056/NEJMp1306445.

Jena AB et al. *The prevalence and nature of postinterview communications between residency programs and applicants during the match.* Acad Med. 2012 Oct;87(10):1434-42.

Kohn, David. *Hopkins Residency Program Loses Accreditation over Labor Rules.* The Baltimore Sun. August 27,2003.
http://articles.baltimoresun.com/2003-08-27/news/0308270239_1_residency-program-hopkins-medicine-program

NRMP Match Communication Code of Conduct.
http://www.nrmp.org/code-of-conduct/

Opel D et al. *Professionalism and the match: a pediatric residency program's postinterview no-call policy and its impact on applicants.* Pediatrics. 2007 Oct;120(4):826-31.

Pease, Allen and Barbara. *The Definitive Book of Body Language.* Bantam, 2006.

Policies and Procedures for Reporting, Investigation, and Disposition of Violations of NRMP Agreements.
http://www.nrmp.org/wp-content/uploads/2014/06/2015-Violations-Policy.pdf

Rogers CL et al. *Integrated plastic surgery residency applicant survey: characteristics of successful applicants and feedback about the interview process.*Plast Reconstr Surg. 2009 May;123(5):1607-17

Swan EC. *Relationship between postinterview correspondence from residency program applicants and subsequent applicant match outcomes.* J Grad Med Educ. 2014 Sep;6(3):478-83.

44776214R00072

Made in the USA
Middletown, DE
15 June 2017